BRAIN UNDER ATTACK

A Resource for Parents and Caregivers of Children with PANS, PANDAS, and Autoimmune Encephalitis

Beth Lambert, MA
Maria Rickert Hong, CHHC, AADP
with Roseann Capanna-Hodge, EdD, LPC, BCN
Lauren Lee Stone, PhD, MS, HHP, BCIH
Jennifer Giustra-Kozek, LPC, NBCC

A Publication Sponsored By:  EPIDEMIC answers

Advanced Praise for Brain Under Attack

"Brain Under Attack is an ambitious undertaking for even the most savvy physicians and scientists regarding the increasing prevalence of neuro-autoimmune disorders (PANS) now facing our children. With statistics indicating that as many as 1 in 200 children are now affected with PANS, parents will again be challenged with a condition of significant disabling severity, with a paucity of resources for assistance. This book provides the reader with the necessary tools to help their affected children via the provision of an excellent overview, case studies, opinions from experts, resources and glossary of terms in a compelling, parent-friendly format, while being current with the latest information available from the field of integrative medicine. An up-to-date laboratory assessment on how to test for PANS is also discussed. Kudos to Lambert and Rickert Hong for bestowing this handbook for parents and practitioners alike!"

—Michelle Perro, MD, Pediatrician and Co-Author of the Bestselling Book *What's Making our Children Sick?*

"Brain Under Attack is a must-have resource! Parents are now armed with all the information needed on how to treat these conditions effectively, combining treating the root cause along with incorporation of integrative modalities. *Brain Under Attack* puts the power back in your hands and allows you to take charge of your family's health in a safe and natural way!"

—Madiha Saeed, MD, Board Certified Integrative Family Physician and Author of *The Holistic Rx*

"This little gem of a book takes a 'Total Load' approach to this elusive illness. Instead of treating those difficult behavioral symptoms and suppressing the immune system with gut-disrupting drugs, learn about possible underlying environmental triggers, infections, and lifestyle factors that are contributing. Read heartfelt parent stories from some who have healed their kids, and find practitioners who will treat you with respect as a member of your loved one's healthcare team. Let this well-researched book be your most helpful guide."

—Patricia S. Lemer, MEd, MS, Bus., Author of *Outsmarting Autism* and *EnVISIONing a Bright Future*

"A lifeline... An empowering and actionable compilation of clinical insights paired with the stories of loving and courageous families rescuing their children, against all odds. *Brain Under Attack* is an important resource for improving our understanding of these conditions and getting children the support they need."

—Kathleen DiChiara, FDN-P, Functional Nutrition Practitioner, Author of *The Hidden Connection* and *Resilience*

Dedication

To the children and families impacted by the
epidemic of PANS and to all of the clinicians,
practitioners and parents working tirelessly to
bring our children back to vibrant health.

TABLE OF CONTENTS

FOREWORD 7

ABOUT EPIDEMIC ANSWERS 11
Epidemic Answers' Mission...11
Acknowledgements 12

INTRODUCTION: MYSTERY ILLNESS 13
Fiona's Story 14

CHAPTER 1: ALL ABOUT PANS, PANDAS
AND ASSOCIATED CONDITIONS 23
What Are the Signs and Symptoms of PANS? 24
How Common Is PANS?..27
What Causes PANS? 28
What Are Some of the Triggers of PANS?...........................32
PANS and Autism..37
Why Does My Child Do That?
What's Happening in Your Child's Brain 38
How Is PANS Treated? 43
A Whole-Child Perspective on PANS 52

CHAPTER 2: STORIES OF FAMILIES IMPACTED BY PANS.. 57
Jenn's Story 57
Pamela's Story 63
Maria's Story 71

CHAPTER 3: HEALING PANS **79**

Epidemic Answers' Four-Step Healing Plan 79

Step One: Take Away the Bad Stuff and
Add Back in the Good Stuff 79

Step Two: Get Help 89

Step Three: Rebalance the Imbalances 91

Step Four: Rehabilitation and Reintegration.............93

I'm Following the Four-Step Plan, Now What?...............95

The Psychological Impact of PANS
on The Child and The Family.. 100

CHAPTER 4: ASK THE EXPERTS **107**

William Lee Cowden, MD.. 107

Elena Frid, MD 116

Tom Moorcroft, DO... 119

Roseann Capanna-Hodge, EdD, LPC, BCN 127

Victoria Kobliner, MS, RDN 131

Lauren Stone, PhD, MS, HHP, BCIH............................. 134

Toby Watkinson, DC.. 136

GLOSSARY.. **145**

A SELECTION OF AVAILABLE RESEARCH **203**

RESOURCES **213**

INDEX... **215**

ABOUT THE AUTHORS **233**

FOREWORD

uddenly Crazy. That was the working title of this book. It came from the mouths of just about every parent whose child has had PANS/PANDAS – an acronym you will soon come to understand thoroughly. I learned all about it because my child was suddenly crazy.

It's a terrifying realization to have about your own child that he or she is suddenly and inexplicably crazy. Facial tics, aberrant behaviors, and mood disorders popping up seemingly overnight. It's an experience that feels torn from the pages of a Stephen King novel when you are living it and is compounded by the shortcomings of our Western medical system where diagnoses can only exist if symptoms can be treated by a pharmaceutical drug. If you are one of the unlucky few to be at the forefront of that curve before a drug has been developed, then you and your "syndrome" will likely be met with some version of disbelief and cynicism. Just ask the sufferers of Chronic Fatigue from 20 years ago, or any of us in the Lyme community. Sadly the medical establishment is of very little use just when you need them most. That's not to say it's all bad - just that there are some serious deficiencies in the system. It's a terrible position for a parent to be in to educate their mainstream medical provider while hoping for a cure from the student! I should know. I am a mom and a medical provider. I've been on both sides.

As a mom of an affected child, I had all the same questions you probably do. How did this happen? Why did this happen? How can it be stopped? As a practicing Physician Assistant, I already knew that the answers didn't yet exist. At least not in the realm of Western medicine. I had to go outside the confines of what I was taught, and more specifically outside the confines of how I was taught to think. Like many parents I had to figure this out on my own. It was stressful and scary and at times it felt hopeless.

You are not alone. Even though it may feel like you are the only one you know with this problem, I can assure you, you are not. As you will soon read, this disorder affects approximately 2% of the children in the U.S., and if my experience as a Lyme mom and clinician tells me anything, it's that we are about to find out that the number is actually much higher. Apart from being a number in an epidemic your struggle is an invitation to another group. We invite you to join the growing legion of people who have found a better way. We are pioneers who have blazed a new trail for the sake of our own children and for this entire generation of children struggling with the unfathomable 50% odds of acquiring a chronic illness. We are a talented and inclusive group who have come together to say "Enough! My child deserves a childhood free from the tyranny of these environmentally-derived disorders!" At Epidemic Answers, we invite you to roll up your sleeves and lock arms as we chart new territory for the sake of our loved ones.

Epidemic Answers started probably where you are now... as a concerned parent looking for answers. Then one became two and they connected to providers already doing this important healing work, and together they built a non-profit resource so no family would have to face this journey alone or have to reinvent the proverbial wheel. Today Epidemic Answers is a robust online repository of credible healing information, webinars, health coaches and a referral network. If you are just getting started, I encourage you to take the Online Training Program, "Healing the New Childhood Epidemics," available to parents as well as professionals to get up this very steep learning curve quickly. It's a self-paced virtual course that educates you about the "why" and "how" of these epidemics.

To learn the "How can it be stopped" piece, well, read on. You have in your hands the combined work of some of the brightest minds at the forefront of the PANS/PANDAS epidemic. These practitioners treat these children –including, in most cases, their own– every single day. They are tireless and well-known advocates for getting to the root cause of these disorders and restoring vibrant health for all children.

This is the book you've been waiting for! We are indebted to the amazing parents and practitioners who have come before us to show us the way and grateful to have you along on the journey.

—Jennifer Boyd, PA
   Chair, Epidemic Answers Board

ABOUT
EPIDEMIC ANSWERS

Epidemic Answers is a 501c3 nonprofit organization dedicated to reestablishing vibrant health in our children and ourselves through education, empowerment and prevention.

Epidemic Answers was founded in 2010 by a group of parents and practitioners who were concerned about the escalating number of children impacted by the "new childhood epidemics": autism, ADHD, asthma, allergies, autoimmune disease and more. In 2013 Epidemic Answers merged with Developmental Delay Resources, a trail-blazing nonprofit organization that for over 20 years brought hope and healing to thousands of parents of children with developmental delays. Together these combined organizations have become the leading authority on the healing the "new childhood epidemics." Epidemic Answers supports research, education, and other initiatives aimed at reversing these devastating health trends.

Epidemic Answers' Mission

Epidemic Answers is dedicated to reestablishing vibrant health in our children and ourselves through education, empowerment and prevention. Epidemic Answers inspires change by:

◆ Illuminating the relationship between such prevalent childhood conditions as asthma, allergies, ADHD and autism to the underlying environmental stressors that negatively impact behavior, development and emotional wellbeing.

◆ Connecting families to healing and prevention resources.

- Empowering parents to partner with their healthcare professionals to optimize their family's health.

- Bringing awareness to the next generation of parents about the relationship between their environments and their future children's health.

The Founders, Board of Directors and followers of Epidemic Answers believe that many of these chronic inflammatory and developmental conditions can be reversed through lifestyle modifications and the personalized application of natural, integrative and whole-child healing approaches. This book reflects this fundamental philosophy and is meant to introduce parents of children with PANS/PANDAS and autoimmune encephalitis to the many healing possibilities.

ACKNOWLEDGEMENTS

This book was written as a collaborative effort with the input, advice and support of many people. The authors would like to thank the following people: Patricia Spear Lemer, MEd and Jennifer Boyd, PA for offering their expertise and editing skills; the Epidemic Answers Board of Directors for providing support and encouragement for this project; the clinical experts who were interviewed for this book including: Dr. Lee Cowden, Dr. Elena Frid, Dr. Lauren Stone, Dr. Roseann Capanna-Hodge, Victoria Kobliner, Dr. Tom Moorcroft, Dr. Toby Watkinson. Most of all, we would like to thank the families who have shared their stories and their hope with us all.

INTRODUCTION
MYSTERY ILLNESS

For all of the deep medical knowledge and technology available in the modern industrial world, it seems hardly possible for a new mystery disease to emerge. And yet, a strange mystery epidemic is sweeping through the youth of industrialized nations, one that is deeply troubling and very poorly understood by the conventional medical community.

This is the PANS epidemic. PANS stands for **P**ediatric **A**cute-onset **N**europsychiatric **S**yndrome (PANS). PANS is an umbrella term which includes diagnoses such as PANDAS, PITANDS, AE and other acronyms (that we will discuss later), all of which describe a condition marked by concerning psychiatric and physical symptoms that almost always appear suddenly. We almost titled this book "Suddenly Crazy" because this is how so many parents describe their experience with this condition. "One day my child was fine, the next day she was 'suddenly crazy.'" It is a horrifying experience for many families and incredibly isolating as few pediatricians have ever heard of, and even fewer know how to treat, this confounding condition. While it is often understood to be a "psychiatric" diagnosis and therefore best addressed through pharmacological, cognitive and behavioral therapies, it is rather an autoimmune medical condition with prominent psychiatric symptoms.

So many parents find themselves watching in horror as their beautiful, "healthy" and typical child descends into the shadows of what appears to be a strange new mental illness. This book is meant to serve as a guide for these parents, a starting place to better understand a condition that is increasingly prevalent, often misdiagnosed, deeply misunderstood, and frightening for impacted families.

You will read stories of families who have "fallen down the rabbit hole" of PANS; some have triumphed over the illness and made full recoveries, and some are slowly emerging from its shadow. You will also hear from experts who treat PANS and who are eager to share their own clinical pearls of wisdom with parents. Finally, this book is filled with definitions, descriptions and references so you can continue to do your own research and bring this material to discuss with your own health care practitioners.

Before delving into the stories, know that children **can** and **do** recover from PANS. It happens all the time. There is hope for healing and it starts with educating yourself and your health care practitioners about this troubling but surmountable condition.

FIONA'S STORY

Before the onset of PANS, Fiona was a typical, happy, seemingly healthy nine-year-old girl. Her parents described her as "bright, happy, funny, confident, independent, kind, outgoing, hard working, and athletic." Then, out of the blue, Fiona began to demonstrate odd and concerning behavior followed by an unwillingness to eat. She soon became very physically ill. The next few months of Fiona's life were harrowing.

THE CHANGES

It all seemed to happen so suddenly, almost overnight. In March of 2016, Fiona developed extreme anxiety, obsessive-compulsive behaviors (OCD), fear of eating, fear of fire, and an unusual but paralyzing fear of glue. She kept thinking that there was glue in her mouth, and she would constantly spit to try and expel the imaginary glue. She wouldn't even swallow her own saliva. She refused to go to school because she had a fear that she would be exposed to dangerous glue there. She also suffered from intense headaches, abdominal pain, numbness and tingling in her feet and hands. Her eyes were always dilated. She had developed a facial tic and lost her handwriting abilities. Fiona's parents were confused, distraught and besides themselves with worry. This was not the daughter they knew.

The onset of her symptoms started about 10 days after she was diagnosed with *Strep* throat, for which she was treated with a 10-day course of antibiotics. In the first days after the symptoms emerged, Fiona was taken to the emergency room (ER) twice. The first time was for severe abdominal pain. Doctors thought the pain might be related to an inflamed or ruptured appendix. It turned out her appendix was fine. The second time Fiona's parents took her to the ER, it was to seek help for her severe head pain. They sent her home from the ER without any answers.

Her pediatrician wanted to diagnose Fiona with anxiety. Her mother contacted a psychologist to explore that diagnosis. The psychologist told her about a diagnosis called PANDAS, which stands for *Pediatric Autoimmune Neuropsychiatric Disorders Associated with Streptococcal Infections.* Fiona was taken back to the pediatrician who agreed with this diagnosis and put her back on antibiotics. He hoped the antibiotics would eliminate the *Strep* infection believed to play a central role in the PANDAS syndrome.

HOSPITAL HOPPING

While on the next round of antibiotics, Fiona's symptoms got worse and worse. She was prescribed a broad-spectrum antibiotic, Augmentin, but this seemed to hurt rather than help the situation. Fiona was taken to The Institute of Living in Hartford, CT to see a psychiatrist as her OCD, anxiety and rages were so intense that her parents and pediatrician didn't know what else to do. She wouldn't eat—she was convinced that there was poisonous glue in her food—and she continued to refuse to swallow her saliva. Her symptoms got so bad that she was admitted for a week at Connecticut Children's Medical Center (CCMC), a highly respected children's hospital, but the doctors had very little experience treating PANDAS. Fiona's parents found themselves calling experts and other doctors all over the state trying to find out best practices for treating PANDAS. Finally, the doctors at CCMC agreed to treat Fiona for PANDAS using a therapy called IVIG—intravenous immunoglobulin—which didn't help at all. Fiona only got worse. Her head pain was extreme to the point that she would feel electric shock sensations in her head and feel as though she couldn't hear. Sleep was nearly impossible. Her parents resorted to driving her around for hours in the evening. The motion seemed to be the only thing that gave her even minor relief. She was afraid of everything, everyone, couldn't stand the sensation of clothes, smells. She was trapped in her sick and terrified body.

Next, Fiona's condition devolved while waiting for lab results from an immunologist specializing in chronic Lyme disease and PANDAS/PANS. Unable to swallow food, water or therapeutics, she was admitted to Yale Children's Hospital for naso-gastric feeding support. Conflicting opinions led the clinical staff to withhold antibiotics prescribed by the immunologist and other than an MRI and some psychiatric medications, Fiona received no other medical interventions.

The week after discharge Fiona received yet another MRI with no findings for the severe and ongoing head pains. Her parents took her to Georgetown to see a well known neurologist who treats children with PANDAS, and Fiona was admitted to the MedStar Georgetown University Hospital. In the hospital, Fiona was given high-dose steroid treatments to treat the significant inflammation driving her symptoms. It was a complete disaster—they made her much worse.

During their hospital stay at MedStar Georgetown University Hospital, the lab test results finally came back from the immunologist revealing extremely high levels of *Strep*, Lyme *(Borrelia)*, *Bartonella*, and *Babesia*, all microbes (believed to be tick-borne). The immunologist told Fiona's parents that her levels were some of the highest he had ever seen.

Fiona was seen by an Infectious Disease specialist at Georgetown. He dismissed the results as not valid and refused to give her antibiotics as prescribed even after speaking with the immunologist. Without much hope or help, Fiona was discharged from Georgetown for "acute worsening of symptoms" and was given anti-psychotic medications.

Fiona was taken back to the immunologist in Connecticut again. At this point she was terribly sick. Physically, she had lost so much weight and was skin and bones. Mentally she was very unstable. The immunologist was extremely worried for Fiona's life and sent her for a second opinion that same day with another well-known pediatric doctor who is a pioneer in tick-borne illness treatment in Connecticut. This doctor and the immunologist conferred during the appointment and, recognizing the deteriorating and extremely critical state of Fiona's health, sent the family to a local hospital in Connecticut for an outpatient feeding tube procedure the next morning so she could receive antibiotics and nutrition.

Fiona had a rage so severe while waiting for the feeding tube procedure that the head of Pediatrics at the local hospital would not allow her to be admitted for the procedure because he deemed it "too complicated." She was then transferred by ambulance to another hospital that was allegedly better equipped for complex medical situations. At this hospital, Fiona and her family had to wait two more days to finally receive a stomach feeding tube. This visit turned into a five-day hospital stay where the infectious disease doctor in the hospital also refused to let her receive antibiotics and didn't give any credence to her lab results.

Once she was released from the hospital and started receiving antibiotics prescribed by her immunologist through her feeding tube, she seemed to gradually improve. It was extremely hard on Fiona's family. Her mother had to stop working for two months and her whole family, including her 11-year-old brother, struggled to deal with the emotional toll of watching Fiona suffer so much. The costs associated with caring for their daughter were racking up, as most of the doctors who were actually able to help Fiona were "outside the box" doctors who don't take insurance.

THE LOWEST LOW

Fiona's mother describes the worst and most traumatic time during this period of hospital hopping.

"The lowest low was between the MedStar Georgetown University Hospital & Maria Fareri Children's Hospital stays, when the neurologist in DC who had saved so many other children seemed to give up on us and never contacted us again. When I finally heard from the neurologist's office, they told me we had left Georgetown AMA (Against Medical Advice); however the doctor on the floor at Georgetown had discharged us for "acute worsening of symptoms" after at least three days of the high-dose steroid treatment, psychotropic medications, and Fiona worsening. We asked them to check our discharge papers but they didn't have a copy, and no results of bloodwork taken while at Georgetown and sent to Mayo to confirm the Bartonella results. We never heard from them again. Our daughter was so mentally and physically ill and raging, and she was suffering terribly, scared and skinny. Our son was so troubled and scared, and it just seemed like Fiona was never going to get better. Nobody would listen except for the immunologist who saved her."

REFLECTIONS ON THE TRIGGER

According to Fiona's parents, the acute *Strep* seemed to be the first trigger for Fiona's symptoms. They believe it somehow caused infection-induced encephalopathy because her immune system was already so compromised. They suspect her immune system was already so taxed because she had been fighting at least three tick-borne infections for at least two years prior: Lyme, *Bartonella* and *Babesia*. For the first 18 months of her recovery, while greatly improved, she still experienced some symptom flares whenever her immune system had an extra burden as with a cold virus, allergies, or another type of infection.

STEADILY IMPROVING

After Fiona had the feeding tube placed and was steadily receiving antibiotics and enteral nutrition, her symptoms began to gradually improve. Fiona's parents feel very strongly that antibiotics worked and saved her life. IVIG didn't work because the infections from tick-borne illnesses were still raging in her body and IVIG wasn't enough. Antipsychotic medications were heavily prescribed by the hospitalists in the beginning, but they didn't help at all. They may have quieted some of the symptoms a bit, but they made her tired, and she was always terrified and in pain.

After many months of trauma in and out of hospitals and conventional doctors' offices, Fiona began working with an integrative doctor and a nutritionist who commonly see children with PANS/PANDAS. After further investigation by this doctor, Fiona's family learned that she had many common nutritional deficiencies and other vulnerabilities that made her more susceptible to the impact of the infections. She has a common genetic variance, MTHFR (a gene variance that impacts how the body uses folate, other B vitamins, and amino acids) which could impact her ability to detoxify, and she also demonstrated evidence of significant mitochondrial dysfunction. She started taking nutritional supplements such as carnitine, vitamin D, a thyroid medication and other supports aimed at building up her immune system.

Fiona still uses a feeding tube for some medications she has trouble taking orally (she was on four antibiotics for 18 months and still taking two antibiotics daily as of this writing), and multiple nutritional supplements but she has put all of her weight back on and more, weighing 75 pounds—finally a healthy weight for an 11 year old! She was down to 42 pounds at the height of her illness two years ago, age nine.

OTHER HELPFUL SUPPORTS

Fiona used a lot of different therapies to help support her health and to rehabilitate her brain after suffering such traumatic inflammation and injury. Salt foot baths helped the pain in her feet early on, and acupuncture gave her some relief from OCD. Cognitive Behavioral Therapy (CBT) was really helpful to get her past some mental hurdles and habits formed during the acute stages of her illness. She did occupational therapy to help get her balance, hand-writing, and other motor functions back, and she has now begun vision therapy (a behavioral approach that prescribes exercises to help resolve functional vision problems).

THE JOURNEY CONTINUES

Fiona is doing so much better. She was still a bit "off" even 18 months later, in that she would make up stories to compensate for the damage that impacted her short-term memory. She could still feel anxious about food at times when she wasn't at home, and still experienced some sensory issues that could cause anxiety. However, she is now back to her happy, active, social, bright, loving self after months of being trapped in a mind and body that were hijacked by this horrible illness. Her goal now is to help other children suffering with PANDAS.

Fiona's parents feel incredible gratitude for the open-minded and integrative doctors who helped her when no one in the con-ventional medical community could. Fiona's mother reflects on their experiences with medical professionals:

> *"We are so grateful to the immunologist who helped Fiona. So many other doctors who are now on her team had such long waiting lists as there are so many families going through this same terrible struggle, and many of these children don't get help in time and have an even longer, more terrible path to get help."*

LESSONS LEARNED

Hindsight is 20-20. When asked what she has learned on this journey and what pearls of wisdom she could offer to other families in the same situation, Fiona's mother now understands that there are "soft signs" of a compromised immune system that can serve as "red flags" to address before things truly go off the rails. While Fiona seemed outwardly healthy to other people, as a baby she had oral allergy syndrome, poor eating and frequently suffered from hives (even in a lukewarm bath). She was also a poor sleeper as a baby and there were other soft signs that something wasn't right.

Reflections from Fiona's mother:

"The health system is broken. Our children are so immunocompromised for so many different reasons that nobody talks about and parents don't hear about, and we don't know the warning signs. There are so many tests babies should receive (e.g., MTHFR genetic mutation) so they won't be as vulnerable as they grow. Tick-borne illnesses are an epidemic and crisis, and children are being treated for psychiatric illnesses or even institutionalized (this was mentioned to us as an option multiple times) when really it is infection-based! Doctors need to be more open-minded and listen! So many families are struggling, and these children are SUFFERING HORRIBLY as the treatments are so expensive and difficult to find. Families are falling apart. So few understand, and families are so alone. We were just so fortunate that we got on the right path "quickly" compared to so many. It needs to be on billboards & every TV talk show!"

Finally, Fiona's mother's advice to other parents:

*"You need to share your story to find out from other families the doctors that can truly help you. Follow your gut when health providers tell you there are no treatment options or don't seem hopeful. Keep looking for answers. Remember it is the illness, not your child, that may do or say things during rages. Cry when you need to, and don't forget to eat. It takes a village, so ask for help. Remember, the recovery can be so slow so try to take it in baby steps as you reach a new normal. You are not alone. **There is hope.**"*

CHAPTER 1
ALL ABOUT PANS, PANDAS AND ASSOCIATED CONDITIONS

C hances are you never heard any of these terms until you or someone you love received this diagnosis. And there is a good reason for this. PANDAS, PANS, PITAND, CANS and AE are a related family of relatively new diagnoses. Unfortunately, this is a category of diagnoses that is growing rapidly, especially among children. So, what are these conditions and why are they impacting so many of our children today?

ALPHABET SOUP— WHAT DO ALL THESE LETTERS MEAN?

The medical community has struggled to define and classify these conditions for the last two decades. The names have changed as doctors and researchers have developed a deeper understanding of what exactly these conditions are. You will be seeing a lot of acronyms thrown about, but for now, they all fall into the category of **PANS**, which stands for **P**ediatric **A**cute-onset **N**europsychiatric **S**yndrome, but even that name does not effectively describe or cover the variations of symptoms seen within this syndrome.

Some other terms you will see used interchangeably with PANS include:

PITAND: Pediatric Infection Triggered Autoimmune Neuro-psychiatric Disorders (Allen et al.)[1]

PANDAS: Pediatric Autoimmune Neuropsychiatric Disorders Associated with Streptococcal Infections (Swedo et al.)[2]

AE: Autoimmune Encephalitis

CANS: Childhood Acute Neuropsychiatric Symptoms (Singer, et al.)[3]

These diagnoses vary slightly, but they all share the common feature of sudden onset of acute anxiety, mood variability and obsessive-compulsive disorder/behavior and/or tics.

With PANDAS, the onset of symptoms is often preceded by *Streptococcal-A* (Group A *Strep*) infection ("*Strep* throat"). However, in many cases the children do not have a history of an acute *Strep*-throat infection.

When this syndrome of symptoms was first identified, the terms PITAND and PANDAS were readily used. The term PANS (Pediatric Acute-onset Neuropsychiatric Syndrome) also came into use shortly thereafter to describe a more generalized syndrome. Autoimmune Encephalitis is a diagnosis more commonly found in adults, but the syndrome is quite similar to PANDAS and PANS. PANS includes not only PANDAS and AE but also diagnoses such as Lyme disease, OCD (Obsessive-Compulsive Disorder) and ODD (Oppositional Defiant Disorder) where there are perseverative and compulsive components to the condition. For our purposes, we will be referring generally to **PANS** which is the broader, and more inclusive, diagnostic label.

WHAT ARE THE SIGNS AND SYMPTOMS OF PANS?

We almost titled this book, "Suddenly Crazy," because that is how so many parents describe their child's primary symptoms. It describes that feeling of shock that a parent experiences when

---

1 https://www.ncbi.nlm.nih.gov/pubmed/7896671
2 https://www.ncbi.nlm.nih.gov/pubmed/8988969
3 http://www.jpeds.com/article/S0022-3476(11)01214-5/fulltext

their typical child exhibits strange, new and disturbing behavioral symptoms that seem to come out of nowhere.

Many symptoms are associated with PANS; in 2010 a working group at the NIH (National Institutes of Health) created a list of common symptoms to help clinicians identify PANS and associated disorders:

I. *Abrupt, dramatic onset of obsessive-compulsive disorder or severely restricted food intake*

II. *Concurrent presence of additional neuropsychiatric symptoms, (with similarly severe and acute onset), from at least two of the following seven categories:*

1. *Anxiety*

2. *Emotional lability and/or depression*

3. *Irritability, aggression, and/or severely oppositional behaviors*

4. *Behavioral (developmental) regression*

5. *Deterioration in school performance (related to attention-deficit/hyperactivity disorder [ADHD]-like symptoms, memory deficits, cognitive changes)*

6. *Sensory or motor abnormalities*

7. *Somatic signs and symptoms, including sleep disturbances, enuresis, or urinary frequency*

III. *Symptoms are not better explained by a known neurologic or medical disorder, such as SC [Sydenham chorea].*[4]

Many times, children presenting with these symptoms can be very sick and are often misdiagnosed with psychiatric conditions due to the severity of their behavioral symptoms. Unfortunately, this can delay proper treatment of what is truly a medical condition. In fact, many conditions believed to be "psychiatric" or "all in the head" have their roots in a body that is deeply out of balance physiologically or excessively burdened with environmental

---

4 https://www.ncbi.nlm.nih.gov/pmc/articles/PMC4340805/

stressors (such as toxins, infections, electromagnetic stressors, emotional stress and more). Following are some of the specific symptoms that parents commonly report as suddenly emerging in their children:

- OCD or obsessive compulsive thinking and behaviors

- Excessive anxiety, especially separation anxiety

- Depression

- ODD or oppositional defiant disorder

- Tics:
  - Hair pulling
  - Eyelash pulling
  - Motor tics such as shoulder shrugging or blinking/winking, jerking
  - Repetitive or compulsive coughing or throat-clearing when not sick

- Excessive and/or lengthy temper tantrums

- Rage

- Mood swings or emotional lability

- Behavioral regression including baby talking, crawling or other toddler-like behaviors

- Developmental regression such as losing the ability to write

- Sensory processing difficulties

- Sleep problems

- Gastrointestinal pain

- Bedwetting

- Severe food restriction

- Spitting, biting, kicking

- Barking, yelling or other verbal abnormalities

- Anorexia

- Decline in handwriting skills
- Decline in math skills
- Hyperactivity
- Inability to concentrate
- Hallucinations
- Head banging
- Aggression (physical and aggressive talk)
- Refusal to go to school
- Increased desire to be left alone
- Seizures

How Common Is PANS?

- Recent statistics indicate that roughly one in 200 children in the United States is affected with PANS. Many experts report that this is a low estimate and PANS may affect more than 2% of children.[5]
- In the United States, it is estimated that between 2%-4% of children have OCD and about 138,000 have Tourette Syndrome.[6][7]
- In addition, 1.5 million American children are diagnosed with anxiety, phobias, OCD and/or bipolar disorder.[8]

Children diagnosed with PANS are typically between one and thirteen years of age, with 60% of diagnoses for children between the ages of four and nine. Increasingly, PANS is now being identified in adults as well.

A Word about Encephalitis

Essentially, within <u>all</u> of these diagnoses, there is encephalitis, or inflammation of the brain. A child with this type of brain inflam-

5 https://www.sciencedirect.com/science/article/pii/S0149763417305833
6 https://www.ncbi.nlm.nih.gov/pmc/articles/PMC3263388/
7 https://www.cdc.gov/ncbddd/tourette/data.html
8 https://www.nimh.nih.gov/health/statistics/bipolar-disorder.shtml#part_155460

mation may never develop certain skills or may lose motor skills and/or the ability to speak, similar to an adult who has had a stroke. Autism and PANS are closely related and as many as two thirds or more of children with autism also have a diagnosis of PANS.[9] Both autism and PANS feature some form of encephalitis, and auto-antibodies to brain tissue are common features of both conditions.

Encephalitis is increasingly common in children and babies today. An increase in a child's head-circumference percentile, especially in the first year of life, can actually signal encephalitis to an astute clinician. The science journal *Nature* pointed this out by stating that "brain volume overgrowth was linked to the emergence and severity of autistic social deficits."[10]

What Causes PANS?

When asked what causes PANS (and associated conditions), most physicians (if they have even heard of PANS—many have not) will tell you that the cause is an autoimmune reaction to an infection (usually *Strep*). But this doesn't explain why some people who experience infection with microbes like *Strep* experience autoimmunity and others do not. It also doesn't explain the fact that this condition is new. Where were all the children with PANS thirty years ago? *Strep* infections are not new. There is currently a lack of true consensus within the medical community as to why some people develop an autoimmune response and others do not. Increasingly, researchers and integrative clinicians who treat these conditions believe that there are multiple factors working in concert to make a child vulnerable to the development of PANS.

First, some believe that children who develop these conditions are already immunocompromised to some degree. This immunocompromised status is subtle and does not fit the criteria for classic immunodeficiency disorders such as CVID, SCID, AIDS or similar. Nonetheless, the children who develop PANS have many signs of a severely dysregulated immune system. Some of the physiologi-

9 http://www.nepans.org/panspandas-info.html
10 Hazlett, H.C., et al. "Early brain development in infants at high risk for autism spectrum disorder". Nature, 542, 348–351 (16 Feb 2017).

cal vulnerabilities commonly seen in children that can lead to a dysregulated, weakened or compromised immune system include:

- Nutritional deficiencies
- Gut dysbiosis/intestinal hyperpermeability ("leaky gut"), often associated with antibiotic use or toxin exposure
- Toxic body burden
- Excessive "allostatic load" or "total load" of stressors on the body (more on this following)
- Lack of outdoor exposure/natural sunlight (often identified as vitamin D deficient)
- Genetic and epigenetic vulnerabilities

What many clinicians hypothesize is that a **compromised immune system** compounded with **breaches to the blood-brain barrier (BBB)** and **concurrent infection with pathogens/toxic exposure** ultimately results in a PANS-like syndrome of symptoms.

Immune system vulnerability + BBB Breach + Pathogens/ Toxic Exposure = PANS

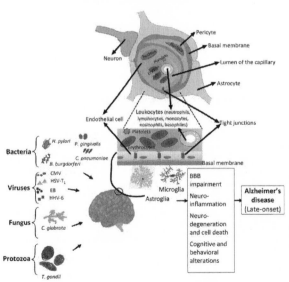

The blood-brain barrier is a protective network of blood vessels that keeps certain things like toxins and pathogens out of the brain. Importantly, the blood-brain barrier also keeps out antibodies. In PANS, however, a breach to the blood-brain barrier allows antibodies into the brain. If the antibodies are targeting brain tissues, receptors and cells, then this breakdown of the barrier is problematic. This allows the immune system to actually start attacking the brain itself.

Source for image[11] Klein TA, Ullsperger M and Danielmeier C (2013) Error awareness and the insula: links to neurological and psychiatric diseases. Front. Hum. Neurosci. 7:14. doi: 10.3389/ fnhum.2013.00014

BRAIN ON FIRE

Neuroinflammation follows this breach as it is the body's way of trying to clear the toxins, pathogens, immune cells and associated debris from the brain. Many of the symptoms seen in PANS/PANDAS are a direct result of this neuroinflammation.[12] Neuroinflammation is also at play in other mood, behavioral, cognitive and psychiatric conditions including depression, bipolar disorder, autism, ADHD, Parkinson's, Alzheimer's disease and more. The discovery that many "psychiatric" conditions involve significant neuroinflammation has been one of the most significant findings in the field of psychiatry in recent history.[13] [14] Children with PANS are really experiencing encephalitis and brain inflammation, and they need to be treated for this medical condition. Their brains are on fire.

A PRIMER ON PANS AND THE IMMUNE SYSTEM

The immune system is a collection of cells, tissues and organs that work together to protect the body from foreign substances called "antigens." Antigens can be microbes and/or toxins, such as:

◆ Bacteria

◆ Parasites

◆ Viruses

◆ Fungi

◆ Pesticides

---

11 https://www.ncbi.nlm.nih.gov/pmc/articles/PMC5476750/figure/F2/
12 https://www.sciencedaily.com/releases/2017/01/170118145937.htm
13 https://www.ncbi.nlm.nih.gov/pmc/articles/PMC5497139/
14 https://www.ncbi.nlm.nih.gov/pubmed/12965267

- Carcinogens

- Mycotoxins

- Heavy metals

- Mold

- Endocrine disruptors

Lymphocytes are small, white blood cells that do the work of the immune system. There are two main types of lymphocytes: B lymphocytes ("B cells") and T lymphocytes ("T cells").

- B cells mature in the bone and are the equivalent of pedestrians jumping up and down outside a burning building yelling, "FIRE! FIRE!" The B cell's job is to "draw attention to the burning building."

- T cells mature in the thymus and are the equivalent of the firefighters who organize and put the fire out.

In immune disorders such as PANS there is an over-proliferation of B cells (the ones yelling "FIRE! FIRE!) and not enough T cells (the ones that stop the screaming or organize how to put out the fire). This is why we talk about one having a "brain on fire."

AUTOIMMUNITY

In a healthy immune system, lymphocytes are able to recognize the difference between "self" and "non-self" cells, attacking non-self cells to eliminate invaders/toxins. In autoimmune disorders such as PANS, the immune system attacks and destroys its own tissues. Autoimmunity means that at some point, the immune system became dysregulated, or its normal "checks and balances" became ineffectual.

Many theories exist as to why autoimmunity develops. One argues that the ecology of bacteria and other components of the microbiome in the gastrointestinal tract and around the body have become imbalanced, much like a polluted pond might become overgrown with harmful algae. This imbalance can be due to diet, antibiotics, toxins and more. When this imbalance in the microbiome occurs, the immune system cannot function properly. If certain gut bacteria, whose primary job is to regulate the immune system ("checks and balances"), are either missing or insufficient, a whole cascade of problematic events occur. Without the proper balance of bacteria in the gastrointestinal tract, the gut lining can become "leaky," allowing microbes, cells, undigested food particles and more to leak into the circulatory system, triggering an immune response or inflammation. Therefore, no matter what autoimmune disorder your child may have—PANS, PANDAS, autism, arthritis and more—healing the gut and balancing the microbes that live there is of utmost importance.

INFLAMMATION

In a healthy individual, immune cells congregate at the site of an infection. Cytokines are immune cells secreted by cells to regulate immune response. Cytokines include interleukins, interferon, tumor necrosis factor and more. When the body is overwhelmed by toxicity, or when a leaky gut allows foreign particles into the circulatory system, cytokines are activated in multiple parts of the body, which can lead to systemic inflammation. High cytokine activity and high inflammation are a hallmark of PANS, PANDAS, as well as autoimmune disorders, autism, ADD/ADHD and Sensory Processing Disorder.

WHAT ARE SOME OF THE TRIGGERS OF PANS?

While it is understood that PANS doesn't really develop out of thin air because the vulnerability has been building over time, it is believed there are certain environmental variables that can serve as the "straw that broke the camel's back." Consider this analogy: Imagine your child as a rain barrel and that stressors of all types (emotional, chemical, physical, and others) are like individual drops of rain falling into that barrel. The barrel (your child) slowly fills with water over time. As each additional drop of water (stressor) is added to the barrel, there comes a point when that barrel cannot accept any more water. Children who develop PANS are typically at their tipping point and then they encounter a trigger, or series of triggers, that push them over the edge. This is why PANS is "acute-onset" or seems sudden, although there may have been overlooked "soft signs" such as chronic constipation, acid reflux, eczema or food allergies/sensitivities from early on. It is important to note that these triggers can also lead to flares, where you will see repeat occurrences of psychiatric or neurocognitive symptoms.

Additionally, the mode of disruption to the blood-brain barrier may impact the distribution of antibodies in the brain, and consequently the types of symptoms that are expressed.[15] In other words, if the antibodies aggregate or concentrate in the temporal lobe, an area associated with short-term memory, this may impact a child's ability to concentrate or stay focused on a task.

Among the many triggers believed to be common in children who develop PANS are:

◆ **Traumatic Brain Injury (TBI) or Concussion.** TBI or concussive head injury opens the blood-brain barrier and causes inflammation in the brain. A child who is already dealing with an infection, or series of infections, or a toxic body burden will find that the opening of the blood-brain barrier and neuroinflammation may allow circulating pathogens and toxins to settle into the inflamed or activated parts of the brain. Parents have reported a reactivation of PANS symptoms in their child following a concussion or other head injury.[16]

◆ **EMF (Electromagnetic Field) Exposure, Dirty Electricity**. Like a TBI or concussion, exposure to strong EMR (electromagnetic radiation) or EMF can also contribute to blood-brain-barrier permeability.[17] [18] Electromagnetic radiation can come from many sources including cell phones, ultrasounds, WiFi and wireless routers, cell phone towers, microwave ovens, cordless phones, SmartMeters, high-ten-

---

15 https://www.ncbi.nlm.nih.gov/pubmed/19668249
16 Dr. Roseann Capanna-Hodge, NEPANS Conference November, 2017
17 https://www.ncbi.nlm.nih.gov/pubmed/25598203
18 https://www.ncbi.nlm.nih.gov/pubmed/24113318

sion powerlines and more. Some parents have reported an increase or relapse in their child's condition upon the installation of stronger WiFi networks into their homes (e.g., 5.0 GHz vs 2.4 GHz).

◆ **Altered Gut Microbiota and Antibiotics.** Exposure to antibiotics can serve to trigger PANS on multiple levels: First, antibiotics disrupt gut-microbe populations which are critical for proper immune function. There is now a significant body of research on how altered gut microbiota or decreased diversity of gut microbiota can lead to "leaky gut" (hyperpermeability of the intestinal lining) and "leaky brain," (hyper blood-brain-barrier permeability). Certain microbes present in healthy guts are known to modulate the "leakiness" (permeability) of the blood-brain barrier. Think about that the next time you take antibiotics. Children with PANS, like other individuals with autoimmune conditions, tend to have less diverse populations of gut microbes than children without PANS. Disrupted populations of gut bacteria can lead to autoimmunity of many types, not just PANS.[19] A recent study completed by researchers at McMasters University in Canada looked at how low doses of penicillin would impact the brains of mice. The researchers "found that **exposure to low-dose antibiotics did affect the mouse brains—and not just a little.** The antibiotic-exposed mice showed an altered blood-brain barrier and a spike in specific immune-signaling molecules (cytokines) in the frontal cortex. Most importantly, however, **the antibiotics changed mouse behaviour:** the young mice acted differently in social situations and when faced with difficult tasks. They were also more aggressive than the mice with no alterations in their gut microbiota."[20] [21]

---

19 https://www.ncbi.nlm.nih.gov/pubmed/25411471

20 Leclercq S, Mian FM, Stanisz AM, et al. Low-dose penicillin in early life induces long-term changes in murine gut microbiota, brain cytokines and behavior. *Nature Communications.* 2017; 8. doi:10.1038/ncomms15062

21 https://www.ncbi.nlm.nih.gov/pmc/articles/PMC4604320/

◆ **Stress, Emotional Trauma, Chronic Inflammation.** There is mounting scientific evidence that a whole host of "stressors" to the body can directly impact blood-brain-barrier permeability, which can leave children more vulnerable to the onset of PANS-type syndromes. Research published as early as 2011 found that mast-cell (a certain type of immune cell) activation triggered by allergies, emotional stress, or other kinds of "stress" on the body can result in blood-brain-barrier permeability. Dr. Theo Theoharides, author of a study published in the Journal of Neuroinflammation in 2011 describes this very phenomenon: *"...brain mast-cell activation due to allergic, environmental and/or stress triggers could lead to focal disruption of the blood-brain barrier and neuro-inflammation"*[22] Essentially, if your child has allergies, eczema, asthma, an autoimmune disease or other type of chronic inflammation, they may be vulnerable to an onset of PANS.

◆ **Injectable Adjuvants.** Certain adjuvants found in injectable medical products designed to elicit an immune response, or to sterilize or preserve the medication, have been found to disrupt the blood-brain barrier and/or facilitate movement of particles across the blood-brain barrier. Polysorbate 80, found in many of these products, is an example of an additive that can shuttle particles across the blood-brain barrier.[23][24][25] Aluminum, also widely used in injectable medical products to overstimulate the immune system, is shown to impact blood-brain-barrier function.[26][27]

◆ **Viral, Bacterial and Fungal infections.** Viral, bacterial and fungal infections have long been known to disrupt the blood-brain barrier. Post-infectious encephalitis is a commonly

22 https://jneuroinflammation.biomedcentral.com/articles/10.1186/1742-2094-8-168
23 https://www.ncbi.nlm.nih.gov/pmc/articles/PMC4318414/
24 http://www.pnas.org/content/108/46/18837.full
25 https://www.ncbi.nlm.nih.gov/pmc/articles/PMC1167690/
26 https://www.ncbi.nlm.nih.gov/pubmed/2671833
27 https://www.ncbi.nlm.nih.gov/pubmed/18786610

understood type of encephalitis that has been seen with a wide variety of infections including measles, *Campylobacter*, mumps and others that are well documented in the medical literature. Other infections may include cytomegalovirus (CMV), hepatitis B, herpes, bacterial infections such as *Streptococcus, Chlamydia pneumoniae*, molds and mycotoxins.[28] [29] [30]

- ◆ **Chemical and Toxin Exposures.** Many healthcare practitioners specializing in PANS/PANDAS believe that blood-brain-barrier breaches may also be due to exposure to environmental toxins. Such chemicals may include heavy metals, formaldehyde, insecticides, pesticides, solvents such as benzene, heavy cigarette smoke and more. What's more, there is a concern that certain toxins can accumulate in cells and tissues and trigger or exacerbate autoimmunity, even in the brain. Increasingly, there is a body of research that looks at how certain toxins set off a chain-reaction of biological disruptions that result in neurodegenerative and neuroinflammatory conditions. For example, one theory postulates that when an individual is exposed to glyphosate (a toxic herbicide), the essential mineral manganese can accumulate in the basal ganglia of the brain stem (more on this later) contributing to movement disorders like Parkinson's, tics and Tourette.[31] Glyphosate is found in the weed killer Round-up and is one of the most widely sprayed herbicides in the world. Glyphosate contamination is found in the vast majority of processed foods.[32] Especially in wheat...

- ◆ **Wheat.** Ever wonder, "what's with wheat?" Research is now bearing out that eating wheat could potentially trigger intestinal permeability and blood-brain-barrier permeability.[33]

---

28 https://www.ncbi.nlm.nih.gov/pmc/articles/PMC3367119/
29 https://www.hindawi.com/journals/mi/2016/8562805/
30 http://www.tandfonline.com/doi/abs/10.1080/21688370.2016.1142492
31 https://www.ncbi.nlm.nih.gov/pmc/articles/PMC4392553/
32 https://www.ncbi.nlm.nih.gov/pmc/articles/PMC4392553/
33 https://www.ncbi.nlm.nih.gov/pmc/articles/PMC4517012/

Exposure to wheat/gluten in the intestinal tract stimulates the release of zonulin, a protein that modulates the permeability of the cells of the intestinal tract and is implicated in blood-brain-barrier function. Essentially wheat can contribute to "leaky gut", a precursor to the development of allergies, autoimmunity and other inflammatory conditions. Unfortunately, zonulin can also lead to "leaky brain" and can result in permeability of the blood-brain barrier.[34]

For those wondering why wheat, and why now, consider that wheat is a commodity crop that is most heavily sprayed with herbicides/pesticides such as glyphosate, which is known to disrupt gut bacteria and impact gut permeability. Even if you eat organic wheat that has not been sprayed with pesticides, if you've eaten enough conventionally grown wheat sprayed with pesticides in your lifetime (think of <u>any</u> restaurant you've ever eaten at) your body will have already been sensitized to the herbicides/pesticides on wheat and may reject wheat as a toxin. Your immune system has a memory, and if you've been exposed to a toxin repeatedly (wheat, oats, nuts, corn, or other commercial crops commonly sprayed), your body will begin to respond to any exposure with inflammation. Yes, even if you eat organic wheat.

PANS AND AUTISM

When the autism epidemic truly took off in the early 1990s, few physicians understood autism as a medical condition with behavioral and developmental consequences. Instead, they conceived of autism as a "genetic" condition that was intrinsic, fixed and intractable, telling parents that their child was just "born this way" and that they would always be this way.

Decades of research and pioneering work done by parents, clinicians and children's health advocates has completely turned this

34 https://www.ncbi.nlm.nih.gov/pubmed/20170845

notion of autism on its head. Autism is now understood to be a whole-body condition, with specific physiological imbalances that impact behavior and neurodevelopment. Some of the medical issues identified in autism include: gut dysbiosis, immune dysregulation, cellular toxicity, mitochondrial dysfunction, neuroinflammation and more. What's more, many families have been able to fully reverse their child's autism (or the syndrome of symptoms we call autism) through targeted diet and lifestyle changes combined with personalized therapeutics aimed at addressing the aforementioned physiological imbalances. Put simply, heal the body, and the brain heals too.

Interestingly, the pathophysiology (or "root causes") of autism is very similar to the pathophysiology of PANS. One of the major differences between the two conditions is that children with PANS tend to experience the neuroinflammation (and other medical issues) *after* critical developmental milestones had already been achieved (e.g., speech development, large and fine motor development, sensory integration, etc.). Children who develop autism are often experiencing this devastating neuroinflammation during critical periods of infant and early childhood development (typically in utero and/or within the first few years of life).

Researchers estimate that approximately two out of three children with autism also have a PANS diagnosis.[35] No wonder, as neuroinflammation is a hallmark of both PANS and autism. Additionally, many children with ADHD/ADD and/or Sensory Processing Disorder (SPD) also have PANS, and neuroinflammation is the common denominator. If your child has a diagnosis of ADHD, SPD, autism or PANS, it would be wise to look for ways to quench that "fire in the brain."

WHY DOES MY CHILD DO THAT?
WHAT'S HAPPENING IN YOUR CHILD'S BRAIN

Why does a child tic? Why do they suddenly develop behavior, attention or other psychiatric symptoms? Your child's immune

---

35 http://www.nepans.org/panspandas-info.html

system is literally attacking cells within certain parts of the brain that govern movement (aha! the tics!), emotional function (aha, the rages!), or behavior (got it! The bizarre behavior!). Think about it this way: if your child has a movement disorder (such as tics), you can pretty much guarantee that a portion of their brain that is associated with motor movement (the basal ganglia) is on fire. This is why you will see some variation in symptoms between different children. Some children have cases of PANS that are more involved with motor function, and some cases are more intense behaviorally.

WHICH PART OF YOUR CHILD'S BRAIN IS ON FIRE?

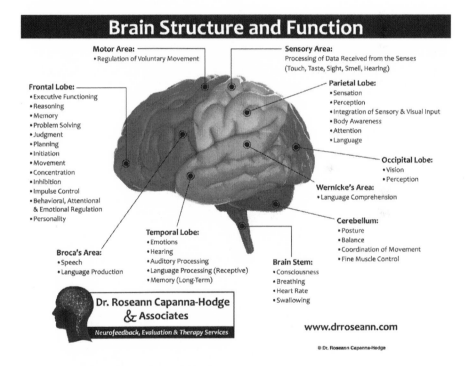

WHY DOES MY CHILD'S IMMUNE SYSTEM ATTACK THE BRAIN?

Buckle up. This is where it gets "science-y." Not interested in the science? That's okay, we'll provide the Cliff's Notes.

Cliff's Notes: The immune system is attacking something in or on the brain cells in an effort to get rid of something that shouldn't be there. In PANS, the immune system is on a "seek and destroy" mission to eliminate anything it perceives as a threat to the body and brain. This might include microbes, toxins or antibodies on the cells of tissues that look similar to certain microbe antibodies or toxins (although researchers are still debating the latter, a theory known as "molecular mimicry.") How did the thing that isn't supposed to be there get there in the first place? See the earlier section on gut and brain permeability. For a variety of reasons, the guards that usually protect the brain were not able to do their job.

So why might a chronic infection with *Strep* cause PANDAS symptoms in my child? Some researchers believe that cross-reactive antibodies created in response to a *Strep* infection actually attack the dopamine receptors in the basal ganglia of the brain because of a blood-brain-barrier breach.

The basal ganglia are a group of nuclei located at the base of the brain and are linked to the thalamus. Basal ganglia have traditionally been associated with movement disorders, such as Huntington's and Parkinson's disease. A feature of PANS is often tics, or movement disorders, so the origin of this symptom makes sense once you know the immune system is targeting something in or around the basal ganglia. In addition to voluntary movement control, the basal ganglia are also associated with procedural learning, eye movements, cognitive function and emotional function.

The basal ganglia are also the site of two dopamine receptors. Dopamine is a neurotransmitter associated with attention, movement and the pleasure/reward centers of the brain.

- ◆ The D1 receptor (Dopamine1) is a direct pathway in the basal ganglia that facilitates movement.

- ◆ The D2 (Dopamine2) receptor is an indirect pathway that inhibits movement.

According to the molecular mimicry theory, when the cross-reactive antibodies associated with *Strep* or other antigens attack the dopamine receptors in the basal ganglia of the brain, it causes a fluctuation in dopamine, which results in OCD, tics and other neuropsychiatric symptoms. Some doctors also refer to this as autoimmune-mediated basal ganglia dysfunction.

While some researchers who subscribe to the molecular mimicry theory believe that the immune system is "misguided" or "confused" and attacking dopamine receptors on the basal ganglia (the antibodies of *Strep* "look like" tissue antigens within the basal ganglia), other researchers believe that some microbes have developed defense mechanisms that allow them to "hide" intracellularly to avoid detection. In this theory the immune system isn't "misguided," it is simply doing its job, attempting to ferret out microbes or toxins hidden within cells.[36] [37] [38]

BRAIN ON FIRE:
ANTI-NMDA RECEPTOR ENCEPHALITIS

A book published in 2013 brought to light another new diagnosis associated with PANS: Anti-NMDA Receptor Encephalitis. The book, titled *Brain on Fire*, by New York Post journalist Susannah Cahalan is a harrowing account of a successful young journalist's descent into psychosis due to Anti-NMDA Receptor Encephalitis. Her experience tracks very closely to the experience of some children with PANS. Anti-NMDA Receptor Encephalitis is very similar to PANS as we have described, only in this case, doctors are able to determine that a patient has developed antibodies to yet another receptor in the brain (NMDA receptors).

The NMDA receptor (N-methyl-D-aspartate receptor) is one of several glutamate receptors found in nerve cells. It is activated when the amino acids glutamate and glycine bind to it. NMDA receptors have been implicated by a number of studies to be strongly involved with excitotoxicity, meaning that when individuals have

36 https://www.sciencedaily.com/releases/2011/01/110126081521.htm
37 https://www.ncbi.nlm.nih.gov/pubmed/26866235
38 https://www.ncbi.nlm.nih.gov/pubmed/16455579

excess quantities of the neurotransmitter glutamate (which can happen by consuming certain foods containing glutamates or when there is a deficiency of glutamate's inhibitory counterpart, GABA (Gamma-AminoButyric Acid, another neurotransmitter), it has an excitatory effect on the brain. Excitoxicity can cause encephalopathy and seizures.[39] Excessive consumption or availability of glutamate (causing excessive stimulation of these receptors) can result in damage to nerve cells. An excess of glutamate that happens due to a deficiency of GABA can be due to gut microbe imbalances, nutrient deficiencies (such as lack of vitamin B_6) and other common causes.[40] Glutamate and its analogs are found in processed foods such as MSG (monosodium glutamate) but also in chemical food additives such as:

- Hydrolyzed vegetable protein
- Soy protein isolate
- Yeast extract
- Gelatin
- Barley malt
- Bouillon
- Natural flavoring
- Artificial flavoring
- Soy sauce

Even natural foods such as tomatoes, bone broth and seaweed may naturally have high levels of glutamate.

In the case of Anti-NMDA Receptor Encephalitis, an individual's immune system is attacking the same receptors that typically receive glutamate, so, in essence, the brain is experiencing excitotoxicity and inflammation in a way that is similar to flooding the brain with excess glutamate. It is unclear why the immune system develops auto-antibodies to this particular receptor, although it has been

39 https://www.ncbi.nlm.nih.gov/pubmed/28870583
40 http://www.pnas.org/content/108/38/16050

hypothesized that certain pathogens like *Mycoplasma* or Epstein-Barr virus may provide a trigger for the autoimmune response.[41]

Researchers continue to uncover the myriad ways that the immune system attacks the brain and brain cells in PANS or other various forms of autoimmune encephalitis. In some ways, it may be irrelevant *which* particular cells are being attacked, when it is more important to understand *why* the body's defense and repair mechanisms are so compromised in the first place that would precipitate this kind of self-attack.

How Is PANS Treated?

In 2017, the PANS Research Consortium (PRC) published treatment guidelines for the management of PANS. Consequently, most families who visit a medical doctor well versed in the treatment of PANS (many are not) will be treated according to the following guidelines:

"Depending on whether a child's symptoms are considered mild, moderate-to-severe, or extreme/life-threatening severity, the treatment varies. For mildly impairing PANS, the most appropriate therapy may be 'tincture of time' combined with cognitive behavioral therapy and other supportive therapies. If symptoms persist, nonsteroidal anti-inflammatory drugs and/or short oral corticosteroid bursts are recommended. For moderate-to-severe PANS, oral or intravenous corticosteroids may be sufficient. However, intravenous immunoglobulin (IVIG) is often the preferred treatment for these patients by most PRC members. For more severe or chronic presentations, prolonged corticosteroid courses (with taper) or repeated high-dose corticosteroids may be indicated. For PANS with extreme and life-threatening impairment, therapeutic plasma exchange is the first-line therapy given either alone or in combination with IVIG, high-dose intravenous corticosteroids, and/or rituximab."[42]

41 https://www.hindawi.com/journals/bmri/2015/643409/
42 Clinical Management of Pediatric Acute-Onset Neuropsychiatric Syndrome: Part II— Use of Immunomodulatory Therapies https://doi.org/10.1089/cap.2016.0148 July 19, 2017

You will notice that these treatment guidelines tend to be pharmaceutically driven and do not include recommendations for diet or lifestyle modifications, which interestingly, seems to be among the most effective treatment strategies based on our collection of families' stories who have reversed or overcome PANS/PANDAS.

CONVENTIONAL/WESTERN MEDICINE TREATMENT OF PANS

For those families who work with physicians unfamiliar with PANS, they will typically see the child's behavioral and emotional symptoms as "psychiatric" and treat with psychotropic and mood-modulating pharmaceuticals. These may include antidepressant or anti-anxiety medications (Ativan, Paxil, Prozac, Zoloft, Lexapro, Xanax, Klonopin, and others). In many cases, children will be subjected to rounds and rounds of different drugs until the doctors and parents find anything that helps. Many parents have found this approach to be a dead end and have often found pharmaceutical approaches to worsen the child's symptoms over the long term. These may be the "easiest" tools, but they are also the least effective and potentially most dangerous for the children involved.

It is important to know that many antidepressants have a "black box" warning against use in children because they can increase the risk of more aggressive behavior and suicide ideation.

More forward-thinking Western medical doctors believe that PANS and PANDAS are typically triggered by a pathogenic infection and/or acute environmental toxic assault.

To that end, treating physicians are often interested in "killing the causative agent" or suppressing inflammation and typical treatment may include:

ANTIBIOTICS

Although a 14-day course of beta lactam antibiotics (penicillin, amoxicillin, etc.) is a typical prescription, many parents do not see improvement on antibiotics until a child has been on them for several weeks or months. Many children require multiple rounds of, or even cocktails of, different antibiotics and some stay on antibiotics for years.

Recent research, however, has shown that antibiotics severely alter, often permanently, the microbiome in the gut, which is where most of the body's immune system is headquartered.[43] [44] [45] In essence, giving antibiotics may "win the battle, but lose the war" because they can alter the body's immune function and can cause "gut dysbiosis" or an imbalance in the bacteria in the gut. Many times this leads to an overgrowth of opportunistic bacteria or fungus in the gut, such as *Candida albicans*, which can further suppress the immune system and lead to an additional immune burden from fungal waste products.[46] What's more, antibiotics only work against bacterial infections, so they won't help in the case of viral, parasitic or fungal infections that trigger PANS symptoms, and antibiotics impair one's ability to detoxify chemicals or other environmental stressors.

STEROIDS AND NSAIDS

Both steroids and Non-Steroidal Anti-Inflammatory Drugs (NSAIDs) have been documented to reduce symptoms in children with PANS and PANDAS, which is a clue that inflammation is part of what's behind the child's symptoms. However, long-term use of either of these kinds of pharmaceuticals is hard on the body and can cause strain on the liver's detoxification process as well as lead to further intestinal permeability and nutritional deficiencies, thereby potentially leading to additional symptoms further on down the road.[47] In addition, steroids can suppress the immune system and disrupt the microbiome in the gut, which can lead to more symptoms later on. Many parents find that NSAIDs can be an effective short-term tool to reduce inflammation and pull a child out of a behavior crisis.

---

43 https://www.ncbi.nlm.nih.gov/pubmed/29562949
44 https://www.ncbi.nlm.nih.gov/pubmed/29517178
45 https://www.ncbi.nlm.nih.gov/pubmed/29459310
46 https://www.ncbi.nlm.nih.gov/pubmed/26442855
47 https://www.ncbi.nlm.nih.gov/pubmed/29221664

IVIG

Intravenous Immunoglobulin (IVIG) treatment is used when a child does not respond well to antibiotics, steroids or NSAIDS because the immune system is severely compromised. IVIG is a blood product containing pooled immunoglobulins (a protein that fights infection) from as many as a thousand donors or more! Immunoglobulins bind to foreign substances so the immune system can find and destroy the foreign substances. IVIG therapy floods the body with donor antibodies, which is kind of like borrowing other people's antibodies to help the child's body fight off infection. IVIG also helps to up-regulate regulatory T cells, thereby improving immune function.

Some children do respond very well to IVIG for relief of their symptoms. Others can have no response or can even experience a worsening of symptoms. IVIG is very expensive, and many insurance companies do not cover it. In addition, one round of treatment may not be enough, especially if the child relapses. There is also a risk in using IVIG just as there is a risk in using any blood products. There is always the potential for contamination as well as any unknown consequences resulting from combining the immunoglobulins of a thousand or more different donors.

PLASMA APHERESIS

Plasma apheresis is rarely used but since it may be offered as a treatment in a hospital setting, it warrants discussion. In a plasma apheresis treatment, the child's blood is collected by a machine, which separates the plasma, red cells and platelets and returns the red cells and/or platelets back to the donor. Some children do respond well to this treatment, but it is expensive and invasive, so Western medical doctors typically reserve it for treatment of children who are severely affected by PANS or PANDAS.

INTEGRATIVE MEDICAL OR "LYME-LITERATE" APPROACHES TO TREATMENT

In some clinics, especially those run by "Lyme-literate" doctors or those who practice functional or integrative medicine, there is a focus on supporting the body's ability to fight infection (by correcting nutritional deficits, microbiome imbalances or metabolic issues) while simultaneously looking for ways to eliminate easily identifiable infections.

These practitioners tend to test for infectious microbes that can be identified through blood work. The most common microbes believed to be involved in the development of symptoms include, but are not limited to:

◆ *Mycoplasma pneumoniae*

◆ Group A *Streptococcus*

◆ *Borrelia burgdorferi*

◆ *Babesia*

◆ *Bartonella*

◆ Varicella virus

◆ Influenza virus

◆ Epstein-Barr virus

◆ Herpes simplex virus

There are likely many, many other infectious or pathogenic microbes implicated in the immune response and neuroinflammation seen in PANS. Because scientists and clinicians have found extremely high levels of these infectious agents in PANS patients, there is a tendency to see those agents as the *sole* cause of the syndrome. A focus solely on the infectious agents, however, overlooks the vulnerability that pre-existed the infection in the child. In other words, why did this particular child succumb to the infection, neuroinflammation and sequelae when another exposed child did not? A strategy of only going after a particular set of microbes can be like playing "whack-a-mole," once you get one, another one pops up, and you can never get ahead of the vicious cycle. PANS is not just a function of exposure to infectious agents, but also a function of a weakened or vulnerable system that attracted the infections and/or struggles to overcome the infections.

COMMON TYPES OF TESTING FOR PANS

A physician who believes infections to be a central part of PANS may choose to have blood tests performed on your child, such as:

◆ **Serum ASO titer** (Anti-Streptolysin O): This is a test looking to confirm the presence of *Strep* antibodies that are produced between one week to one month after the onset of an infection.

◆ **Serum ASDB titer** (Anti-Streptococcal DNase B): This is another test looking to confirm the presence of *Strep* antibodies. This peaks four to six weeks after infection and remains elevated longer than ASO.

◆ **The Cunningham Panel:** This is a series of tests that was developed by Madeleine Cunningham, PhD to help physicians diagnose and treat infection-induced neuropsychiatric disorders. These tests measure circulating levels of auto-antibodies directed against specific neuronal antigens, including:

  • Dopamine D1 receptor (DRD1)

  • Dopamine D2L receptor (DRD2L)

  • Lysoganglioside GM1

  • Tubulin

Put simply, the body is making antibodies that attack the aforementioned brain proteins, and these tests identify if some of these antibodies are present. If they are present (positive test results) concurrent with neuropsychiatric symptoms, then physicians come to the conclusion that the child is experiencing infection-related neuroinflammation. A positive Cunningham Panel is often used to confirm that a child has an autoimmune disease affecting the brain. For many doctors and families the Cunningham Panel has been used to convince naysayers that there is a serious medical condition present and not just some "psychiatric" problem that can be treated with psychotropic medications or cognitive behavioral therapy.

A Word of Caution about Lab Tests

Conventional lab tests are not always reliable. Titers are not always indicative of an infection. With regard to *Strep* testing, titers are often only moderately elevated, or not elevated at all in some children with PANS. According to one study, only 54% of children with *Strep* throat showed an elevated ASO titer and only 45% showed an increase in Anti-Streptococcal anti-DNase B.[48]

In addition, throat cultures frequently result in false negatives because of the technique used in obtaining the specimen, mishandling of the specimen and the fact that the *Strep* bacteria may be harbored in other parts of the body than the throat.

And most importantly, positive lab tests are NOT required for a diagnosis of PANS. A PANS diagnosis is made through a clinical diagnosis of positive neuropsychiatric and/or neurocognitive symptoms.

Testing for Blood-Brain-Barrier Dysfunction

There are some practitioners who use advanced antibody testing to evaluate blood-brain-barrier competence. Patients with neuro-autoimmunity may have high levels of blood-brain-barrier protein antibodies, and clinicians use the following tests to evaluate blood-brain-barrier disruption:

◆ Antibodies to S100-B[49]

◆ Antibodies to occludin

◆ Antibodies to zonulin[50]

Remember: *Because labs are not always reliable, the diagnosis of PANS is truly a clinical diagnosis.* This means that your healthcare provider will base his or her diagnosis on your child's history and symptoms. However, labs can be helpful for confirming a clinician's suspicion about what is going on medically with your child.

---

48 https://academic.oup.com/jid/article/188/6/809/943043
49 https://www.ncbi.nlm.nih.gov/pubmed/27357716
50 https://www.ncbi.nlm.nih.gov/pmc/articles/PMC1866950/

Non-laboratory Methods of Testing

There are many other noninvasive methods of assessing imbalance in the body including infections. Some of these methods are hands-on methods used by skilled practitioners, and some are computerized methods of testing. Following are some testing methods commonly used by integrative or holistic practitioners, most of which have not been rigorously tested for accuracy or reproducibility. Nevertheless, many practitioners and families attest to their usefulness in a clinical setting.

- ◆ **Bioenergetic Assessments** measure energy, electrical conductivity and/or electrical imbalances in the body by utilizing an electronic instrument (Avatar, Zyto, Asyra, Qest4, ART, Biomeridian testing are some common names) to gather information via acupuncture meridians or via bioresonance. Many bioenergetic testing modalities measure electrical conductivity through pressure on acupuncture points. Another way to describe this approach is testing via electroacupuncture. These systems were developed based on the observation that electrical conductance of the body will change when it is exposed to something that triggers a stress response (allergens, toxins, etc.). Some practitioners use bioelectric tools that look for "resonance" in the body, to evaluate the presence of pathogens, toxins or other factors. In this case, the electrical tools send a frequency-based signal to the body (via a conductive material) and interpret the body's response based on whether or not the signal resonates (matches the frequency). These technologies are still in their infancy but are beginning to be studied for their clinical significance.[51] Anecdotally, many families have benefitted from these types of non-invasive assessment tools.

- ◆ **Applied Kinesiology (muscle testing)** is a practice used by many chiropractors and other healthcare practitioners as a way to use the body's natural stress response to help iden-

---

51 https://www.karger.com/Article/FullText/365742

tify various imbalances, deficiencies or irregularities in the body. By testing the strength of certain muscles (or by looking for tension in a muscle or muscle group), the practitioner can gather information about the body. Muscle testing is commonly used to test for sensitivities and intolerances (for which there are no "gold standard" laboratory tests) and for the presence of certain infections. The medical literature is limited on applied kinesiology, due in part to the fact that it is a clinical art that is largely dependent on the practitioner and his/her skill and technique. Regardless, many clinicians use this method with great success, and families report positive outcomes through the use of this tool. While more studies of this method would certainly be welcome, it has proven to be a low-cost, non-invasive and gentle clinical tool for clinicians supporting patients with chronic conditions.

◆ **Intuition and Medical Intuitives:** We have included a section on intuition and medical intuitives in the testing section of this book on PANS because this method is widely used, often successfully, among people who suffer from medical mysteries or unrelenting chronic conditions. Humans are complex, multi-faceted and highly sensitive beings and while science has elucidated so much of what was once unknown about human health, we still have much to uncover.

Human beings all have intuition or an inner sense of knowing. Some cultivate and sharpen this intuition and others flat-out ignore it. In medicine, physicians have been using intuition for millennia, relying on their training but also their gut feelings about what a patient needs or what may be at the root of a particular patient's health challenges. As American medical culture shifted towards preferencing evidence-based practices above all else in the latter part of the 20th century, classic physician intuition became viewed as irresponsible and was widely denigrated by colleagues.

But is the need for evidence wholly incompatible with the use of intuition?[52] [53]

Many families of children impacted by PANS have worked with medical intuitives (or simply physicians not afraid to use their intuition) to help identify some of the root causes of their child's condition. Medical intuitives are individuals who have a heightened attunement to subtle energies or have other ways of receiving information about a patient they are working with.

Because medical intuition varies so greatly from practitioner to practitioner, it has not stood up to rigorous controlled studies. However, an openness to working with a skilled medical intuitive has brought many people answers that they could not get working solely in a conventional medical setting. Perhaps medical intuition should be viewed more openly as a complementary approach to gathering information about health and well-being.

A WHOLE-CHILD PERSPECTIVE ON PANS

Although PANS is often described in terms of an "acute onset" and/or specific microbial infections, it cannot be distilled down to a specific causative factor. Almost invariably, when a child succumbs to PANS, it is usually due to a "perfect storm" of factors. It is almost never just about the infections or the microbes that seem to be plaguing a child's body. In order to develop the syndrome known as PANS, the child's body needed to be vulnerable to the infections and the autoimmunity in the first place.

Following are some of the factors typically contributing to a child's vulnerability to developing PANS:

◆ Environmental exposures to toxins, including pesticides, herbicides, heavy metals, petroleum-based chemicals and many more. Just living in the modern world makes one vulnerable to these exposures.

---

52 https://www.ncbi.nlm.nih.gov/pubmed/9231295
53 http://online.liebertpub.com/doi/abs/10.1089/act.2000.6.331

- Infectious agents, including the microbes identifiable through laboratory testing such as *Strep, Borrelia,* and *Babesia* as well as microbes that cannot yet be easily detected.

- Genetic "fault lines" or vulnerabilities, such as a MTHFR C677T or A1289C variant which makes it more difficult to detoxify. This is a common variation, affecting as much as 50% of people of certain ethnicities.

- Stress, including emotional stress, psychological stress, or any type of physiological stress on the body. Often times people overlook the importance of family stress. Are the child's parents getting along? Did the family recently move? Is one of the child's parents dealing with excessive work or job stress? Was there a recent trauma in the family such as a car accident or a death in the family?

- Nutritional deficiencies where a child lacks critical nutrients required for proper immune function, such as essential fatty acids, vitamin D, zinc, iron, magnesium or others. These nutritional deficiencies are not just for children considered to be "malnourished." In fact, most U.S. children have some, if not many, nutritional deficiencies due to the nutrient-poor Standard American Diet.

- Pre-existing gut dysbiosis or an imbalance/lack of microbial diversity in gut microbes. Gut dysbiosis is very common in children who have a history of frequent antibiotic use. This effect is also multi-generational. If a mother had high exposure to antibiotics throughout her lifetime, she will pass this vulnerability on to her children. Gut dysbiosis is very common in the modern world and can have a profound impact on immune function.

- Poor sleep is a common contributing factor to depressed immune function and toxic build up. The body's immune system is very busy during sleeping hours, detoxifying the body and brain, and rebuilding and repairing damaged tissues. If children do not get enough regular sleep (or if their sleep is interrupted or fragmented due to sleep disorders such as sleep apnea), their immune function will suffer considerably.

◆ Reduced exposure to natural sunlight. Lack of adequate sun exposure can contribute to low vitamin D levels but can also impair energy production, natural sleep and other bio rhythms, and detoxification capabilities.

There is no single cause or agent behind PANS; rather, there are multiple contributing factors that work together in precipitating the disease process. In most cases there was a history of a "loaded gun" (multiple pre-existing vulnerabilities) and a "trigger," something that tipped these vulnerable kids over the edge to develop the symptoms of PANS. That "loaded gun" is what we call the "total load."

TOTAL LOAD THEORY

What makes a child vulnerable to a condition like PANS has to do with their "total load," a term coined by educator and autism expert Patricia Lemer, to describe the total cumulative burden of stressors on the body. "Stressors" is a word used to describe something in the environment or in someone's experience that places excessive stress on the body or requires that the body have resources (nutritional, biochemical, etc.) to meet the challenge. Examples of stressors on the body may include:

◆ Toxic chemicals (including those found in everyday products)

◆ Pesticides, herbicides, fungicides

◆ EMF exposure (from WiFi, cell phones, iPads, SmartMeters, ultrasounds, etc.)

◆ Emotional stress (from a parent deployed overseas, or from the death of a loved one, for example)

◆ Unaddressed vision impairments such as a strabismus or convergence disorder (as vision places an extraordinary drain on a body's resources)

- Junk food
- Microbial infections (this includes persistent infections with molds, fungi, bacteria, and viruses)
- And more.

The accumulation of all of these factors stresses the body, putting it over its threshold for handling stressors, and allowing the disorder to progress. Individually, the human body is well equipped to manage any one of these stressors without showing symptoms of illness or disease. However, experienced cumulatively, the human body begins to break down, especially if the body does not have enough existing resources (sleep, nutrition, movement, downtime, etc.) to handle the cumulative load.

Total load is made worse for children who do not have the biological, emotional or physiological resources to handle this cumulative burden. Some of the things that increase an individual's resilience and ability to tolerate an excessive burden of stressors include:

- Strong emotional ties to others
- Feeling loved, supported, safe and cared for
- Exposure to the natural world (trees, forests, beaches, dirt, fresh air)
- Exposure to natural sunlight
- Adequate daily sleep
- Adequate daily hydration
- Adequate daily nutrition
- Diversity of microbial friends in and around the body (such as gut microbe diversity)
- Regular exercise and movement

MULTI-GENERATIONAL TOTAL LOAD

Every person has a unique "tipping point" as well as his or her own unique path to total load. This total load does not necessarily begin with the child. Scientific research has shown that trans-generational toxins and other stressors or vulnerabilities can be passed down from parents to child. Toxins are passed from a mother to a child *in utero*. Nutritional deficits can even have a multi-generational effect, so that if an individual had a nutrient-poor diet, it can have an effect for several generations. What's more, the child's gut is often (if born vaginally) populated with the same microbes of the mother. If the mother has an imbalance in gut bacteria, then the child is likely to develop a similar imbalance, setting the child up for immune dysfunction.

NOW WHAT?

Now that you have seen that there are a number of different viewpoints on PANS, what causes it and how it can be treated, we would like to bring you the perspective of families who have been there—families who have dealt with a child with PANS and want to share their pearls of wisdom with you. Following these stories, you will find a section on Healing PANS. Our focus has been on finding the families and practitioners who understand what causes PANS, who treat the root causes rather than suppress the symptoms and who believe fundamentally in the capacity of the human body to heal. We have aggregated many types of healing modalities and approaches because no one method is perfect for every person, and each child should be considered on an individual and personalized basis.

CHAPTER 2
STORIES OF FAMILIES
IMPACTED BY PANS

Following are the stories of families that have been impacted by PANS and PANDAS. It is our hope that these stories provide hope and inspiration for families that are looking to heal their children. These families were interviewed by Epidemic Answers in 2017.

JENN'S STORY

"At the end of the school day I received a call from the school nurse that there was something very wrong with Elaina. When I arrived at the school, I see Elaina huddled over on the floor in a ball. She was rocking back and forth. When I brought her home, she started yelling and screaming "I don't know what's wrong with me – I want to kill myself."

How would you describe your child before the onset of PANDAS/PANS/AE? What was she like?

My daughter Elaina, now 10 years old, had always been a beautiful, bright, sweet and happy child. Although slightly anxious at times, she is a wonderful kid, she does well in school, has many friends, is a fantastic dancer with a lot of joy in her eyes and energy in her step. She was always alert and lively, a good learner, physically active with a good appetite.

Did your child have any of the "soft signs" of a pending chronic illness (such as allergies, chronic ear infections as a baby, eczema, dark circles under the eyes, attention issues, constipation, diarrhea, "tummy aches," etc.)?

Interestingly, I had been on the journey to heal my son from autism since 2010 by addressing his underlying immune system, metabolic and digestive issues by healing his gut, correcting for many deficiencies and adopting an organic lifestyle free of pesticides and genetically modified ingredients. I should have listened to my very intuitive daughter when she told me that she was going to write a book titled, "What About Me?" I had always figured it was just jealousy that we were spending so much trying to take care of Evan. I didn't listen. Elaina didn't have the same manifestation of symptoms as her brother and seemed to be meeting every developmental milestone, so I ignored some of the softer signs that she too had a less-than-perfect immune system. From birth, she was never the best sleeper. She had terrible colic, and although breastfed she would get terrible diaper rash and would projectile vomit all the food I was feeding her. She was on prescription antacids at age two months old. She had colic and cried excessively. She only seemed comforted by my touch. She also suffered from dark circles under the eyes and chronic ear infections. She received two rounds of ear tubes. Every time she ate, she complained of having a tummy ache. At age six, she was tested for food intolerances after she became very angry one hour after eating ice cream, and it appeared a pattern was developing after she ate certain foods. In addition, I called her my "virus girl" because she would seem to get Strep throat often and every virus under the sun. While on a Jamaica vacation in April 2015, Elaina was bitten by a mosquito and her eyes became swollen shut. Within a day, she developed a high fever. The resort called for an MD who put her on a steroid and a heavy-duty antibiotic in fear that she contracted a dangerous mosquito-carrying illness. Between the antibiotic and the steroid, I believe that we suppressed her immune system so much that within 24 hours after starting medication, she had the worst outbreak of HSV-2 I had ever seen. Her mouth was completely covered in blisters inside and out, and she was unable to eat without pain; she was so sick. Since then she would get more mild outbreaks when under extreme stress or when her resistance was down.

When did you notice that something neurological was happening with your daughter? Were there any sudden changes that you noticed?

I suspected something was drastically different about Elaina in late February 2017. Seemingly out of nowhere, she started crying inconsolably. When I asked her what was wrong, she told me that she had watched a shark attack video on YouTube the day before. My immediate reaction was one of guilt, that I should be paying greater attention to what she was watching on YouTube. Then I noticed that she could not get the disturbing thoughts or images out of her head despite all my psychotherapy tricks I was pulling out of my bag. I even gave her bilateral stimulation which was an adaptation of Eye Movement Desensitization and Reprocessing (EMDR). It seemed to calm her enough to fall asleep that night, but by the next day she began ruminating about other disturbing things as well. When asked, Elaina said, "I can't make the disturbing thought in my head disappear." She also started complaining of a terrible stomachache which I figured was due to her nervousness or perhaps she had a stomach virus. She had missed so much school already for chronic Strep and other illnesses, and we were leaving on vacation to Disney the following day, so I made her go to school anyway. At the end of the school day I received a call from the school nurse that there was something very wrong with Elaina. When I arrived at the school, I see Elaina huddled over on the floor in a ball. She was rocking back and forth. When I brought her home, she started yelling and screaming "I don't know what's wrong with me – I want to kill myself." I emptied her lunchbox to find that she hadn't eaten her lunch at all. So, I assumed she was just so upset because her blood sugar was low and she was just hungry. When I tried to feed her, she pushed her food away and told me that a voice in her head was telling her not to eat or drink.

How was your child diagnosed? Did you experience any push-back from the doctors you sought out for help?

All of a sudden, all my mommy gut instincts began to kick in. Oh my God, something was seriously wrong with my baby. I started to suspect that she had Strep throat again. I called the school nurse and asked her if Strep was going around again and she replied, "not really – Elaina doesn't have a fever and she isn't complaining of a sore throat." I took her to the walk-in clinic anyway, and I am so grateful I did. My instincts were right. My daughter wasn't developing a mental illness or anorexia - she was Strep positive, and she was developing PANDAS (Pediatric Autoimmune Neuropsychiatric Disorder Associated with Streptococcal infections). I am just so grateful that I knew something about PANDAS from the biomedical community I had the privilege of learning from previously. Knowing what I knew, I probably would have just run to a PANDAS-literate physician first, but we were leaving on a flight the next day, and I wasn't going to mess around with this. I knew how serious it was. I hesitantly accepted the script for amoxicillin and started treating her that night. By day three of the medication, we called the clinic at home and switched her to azithromycin. It appeared she may have developed a resistance to the other. Elaina was in Disney World but wished she was sleeping in bed at home. My daughter, who is typically full of energy, needed to ride in a baby stroller through the parks. She had zero energy to walk. She refused many rides and was experiencing tremendous noise sensitivity. She held her ears and would start crying at the slightest trigger. She was so depressed and was having terrible temper tantrums with aggression. She continued to have obsessive thoughts about the silliest of things. At times, I was afraid that hotel security would come after hearing Elaina screaming uncontrollably. When we returned home, I brought Elaina to her pediatrician for a follow-up Strep test, so that we could document what was happening and so that I could get a referral to see an Ear, Nose & Throat Specialist about a possible tonsillectomy. When I spoke to the pediatrician her response was, "Oh that's an interesting story. Yes, PANDAS is a very controversial topic." Honestly, at this point, I have lost all energy trying to convince the mainstream medical community – what I know to be true. I had been down a similar journey before with my son. And, I knew that if I wanted validation, true answers and real treatment – I would need to go to a doctor of naturopathic medicine (ND) or an Integrative or Functional Medicine MD.

What was the lowest point for you, your child and your family along this healing journey?

Our healing journey through PANDAS and back again wasn't an easy one. Our family's heart began to break as we witnessed Elaina disappear in front of our eyes. The stress it brought to our family was unbearable. To see the pain in Elaina's eyes. To witness the beating of her head on the floor, the refusing to eat and the obvious psychiatric symptoms that were showing up. It saddens her to recall how depressed she felt during that time. To compound issues, she felt so responsible for the way we were all reacting to her. We knew she was sick, but we would lose patience with her at times. The only light at the end of the tunnel was that we felt armed with the best treatments available. Instead of freezing in fear, which is easy to do, we decided as a family that we would learn everything we needed to so she could heal. We were absolutely determined and knew we would succeed. And, Elaina took control of her own treatment, which I believed helped tremendously to bring her back to health.

What therapies did you try? What worked? What didn't work? Which therapies were the most impactful?

After completing one and a half rounds of antibiotics, my first step was to take Elaina to a practitioner that did applied kinesiology. He muscle tested her to determine all underlying pathologies. He discovered that the reason for her chronic recurrence of Strep was due to underlying Lyme disease. Her immune system was tanked. Her adrenals were exhausted, and she had excess yeast in her gut. The practitioner started her on a five-month protocol. She started taking immune-boosting herbs, minerals and vitamins in the form of a chewable tablet called Kindermune by Priority One. She also started taking an adrenal-support capsule, a special ABX Support probiotic by Klaire Labs, a colloidal-silver spray, a detoxification kit and Strep and Borrelia homeopathy by DesBio. Approximately half way through the protocol, I consulted with my naturopathic physician who specializes in homeopathy. She did some blood work to validate what we had learned from the applied kinesiology practitioner. She felt that the nosode remedies were great for helping to drain and excrete the disease but wanted to put Elaina on some constitutional remedies to help with deeper and more profound healing. So, she started her on a series of different remedies by Hahnemann Laboratories. Simultaneously, she began receiving energy healing in the form of craniosacral therapy and reiki. Everything in the healing strategy has the goal of eliminating stress, increasing the energy in her cells and improving her immune system to fight the good fight. Elaina began getting BioRegulation Therapy (BRT) to help her cells better communicate with each other and help restore balance in her body. She also started to see a psychotherapist to help her release all the emotion that she was holding inside. She began to learn that holding negative emotion and self-hatred weakens the body and lowers immune response to illness.

How is your daughter doing now? What do you do to support her in the aftermath of this experience?

Elaina is doing amazingly well. Her mood has dramatically improved. Her noise sensitivity has disappeared. She is the happy and well-adjusted little girl with boundless energy. She is back to the child I have always known. We continue with our organic food lifestyle and continue to support her nutritionally. We give her whole-food supplements, hyperbiotics (Pro-Kids) —a special probiotic designed for inner ear, nose and throat support. She continues to see a therapist, and we watch for any evidence of immune weakening. We do notice if under stress or during periods of exhaustion that she tends to flare a little bit, but now we know exactly what to do to support her.

What is the single most important thing you have learned from being on this healing journey with your child?

TRUST YOUR GUT! You know your child best. Our intuition is our best guide!

PAMELA'S STORY

"My son suffered from a resistant strain of Strep, EBV and CMV simultaneously that caused him to developmentally regress by several years in what seemed like it was overnight."

How would you describe your child before the onset of PANDAS? What was he like?

My son was lively and energetic. He was a happy, carefree, child who was intensively active in school, sports and home with a keen sense of humor.

Those are the words we used to describe how our now 10 year-old was about four years ago (and thankfully is again today). You would never know that he fought a fierce battle to regain his health.

It is scary how quickly life and health can change. It all started the first week of January 2013 when our son who was turning six had a terrible illness and sinus infection, and we had to cancel his birthday party.

What happened to your son? Can you describe how his PANDAS/PANS symptoms emerged?

Like most kids when they are ill, we kept him home for a few days (which was easy as it was the tail end of the holiday break) and then sent him back to school. We don't recall any consequential events immediately following the holiday break. Of course, everyone is slow to recover after the holidays, so perhaps we (his parents, teachers, and coaches) were paying less attention than we would at other times of the year.

About three days after the holiday break, he started eye blinking. Then we noticed new symptoms: shoulder shrugging, throat clearing and head turning, and he started washing his hands 20-30 times per day. About a week later he started talking in baby talk, and his speech was loud and uncontrolled, and he was just talking nonsense. His eyes were constantly dilated, and he started sucking his thumb and being clingy. He even crawled one evening. At that point (and for several more months), he complained of constant head pain even though he had previously shown to have a very high pain tolerance.

Now we were scared. Even his teachers noticed something wasn't right. We were so concerned that we took him to the pediatrician's office four times in two weeks. How could a normal, active, vivacious child turn into this!? Our doctors told us it was allergies, "kids act funny sometimes," it might be Tourette, and then finally the fourth doctor said we needed to do some labwork on him.

Can you remember what precipitated his symptoms? What do you think might have contributed to his condition?

Looking back at our notes, we saw that he had been put on antibiotics the second week of January for a sinus infection and possible Strep throat, even though the doctors never took the time to swab his throat to confirm it was Strep. (I, Mom, also was very sick the following week with what we believe to be the same thing). By the end of February, the labs showed our son had above-normal Strep titers (100-200 range), high CMV (cytomegalovirus) and high EBV (Epstein-Barr virus) as well as many vitamin/mineral levels well out of normal range (both extremely high and low).

His teacher was concerned enough that she asked a fellow parent who was a doctor to reach out to me and help our son. This parent was kind and explained the lab work. At the same time, the fourth pediatrician had given us a diagnosis of OCD and wanted to put our son on OCD/anti-tic medication. While we do believe in Western medicine, we weren't ready to put him on this type of medication without additional specialists, more information and second or third opinions.

How were you feeling during this time?

This was a very scary and lonely time. Many people didn't understand what was happening to our son, and we barely had enough information to understand it ourselves, let alone explain it to others. Many people thought our son was contagious by the way he was acting, but we knew he wasn't. We just didn't know how to explain why and how. About that time, we used every last connection we had to get him into the area Children's Hospital to see a neurologist. Unfortunately the wait was about one month (down from normal three months), which seemed like eternity.

Hour by hour and day by day he was worse, and by February 8th, we decided we weren't going to put up with waiting any longer. His tics were worse, his headaches were debilitating and his personality disappeared. All we saw was a lost child with a blank stare that couldn't understand or communicate what was happening to him. He even had dark thoughts of mortality-both his and those close to him. I made the scary decision, even though I was unsure of how to explain my story, to reach out to the parents support group locally. Thankfully, the founder spoke with me on the phone. She said "You are not alone. You don't know me but please put him on antibiotics, and you have to get his tonsils out" and gave me the name of a doctor that had actually treated hundreds of children all over the U.S. We sent this doctor our son's labwork, and he wanted more updated labwork.

What kinds of treatment did your son receive and how did they impact him?

Within 24 hours of that phone call our son was on cephalexin along with olive leaf extract, multivitamin, a complete omega and round-the-clock Motrin. Within four days of that phone call (February 12th), and each and every day for the next five weeks we saw a calmer child. He was performing well at school but still dealing with the constant eye blinking and headaches, but the life still wasn't in his eyes and his wild sense of humor wasn't back. He also grunted while trying to fall asleep and spent 12-14 hours per day sleeping.

When he wasn't sleeping, he wanted to rest and was tired. This didn't seem right since we used to call him "The Energizer Bunny."

It took about 10 days but around mid-February, the new lab work showed improved vitamin/mineral levels and decreasing EBV and CMV levels. However, the Strep titers were higher and now in the 200-300 range. So he was switched from cephalexin (two teaspoons twice per day) to augmentin/azithromycin (one teaspoon each per day at different times of day), and he improved yet some more.

We were thrilled when we got into the specialist at the Children's Hospital. I still remember thinking he looks too well; this doctor will never believe he has a problem. But he did show enough twirling around and around, hand-washing, and dilated eyes that this doctor believed something had happened and said they could cure him but it would be a long road. This doctor pulled yet another eight vials of blood, had us start a headache log, closely monitored the antibiotics, asked us to schedule a tonsillectomy and remove gluten from his diet. Between these two doctors and the ENT, we felt hope we hadn't felt in a long time. Ten days later, the labwork showed slow and steady increases in his health, and he was on the path to normal levels.

How did you deal with the daily challenges presented by your son's condition?

It is amazing how difficult and monumental things are at the time. I remember thinking there is no way our son will take the antibiotics since they taste terrible. Well, we got through that. I remember him telling me "Mommy, I can't swallow pills." Well, he got over that. I remember holding him down to draw his blood. Later he got eight to nine vials of blood drawn without incident. I remember thinking all our son wants to eat is sugar and carbohydrates and him saying "I'm not going to be gluten-free or have no sugar." Well, we did come to a compromise and gave up gluten, and sugar is only one to two times/week.

Where did your son's treatment go from here?

On May 30, 2013 our son had his tonsils out, and the tonsil microbiology showed Strep resistant to clindamycin and enthromycin. We felt like we had gotten "the enemy." The Children's Hospital Doctor switched our son to Ceftin on June 23rd. While eye tics were minimal, the life in his cheeks came back and so did his humor. The headaches were gone. We were cautiously optimistic and enjoyed a family vacation together (medicine and all).

At this point we were unsure on the best course of action, so we decided to stay the course. Didn't your Grandma tell you "If it ain't broke, don't fix it"? Research and literature showed the length and treatment really depended upon how long the child had been ill before they were treated. While people are still trying to figure out how to classify this condition (similar to rheumatic fever or autoimmune encephalitis), it has been said that those can require years of antibiotics to ward off future infection and reduce inflammation. Both the doctors and we felt good we had caught it within six weeks, but his immune system had a long way to go. We have truly learned how long it takes to rebuild one's immune system.

Meanwhile, we had heard reports of "carriers" and had the entire family's labs pulled. Everyone was normal except me, Mom. That was a serious blow. Turns out I had Strep titers of 500-600 range. I went on and off antibiotics from June 2013 – February 2014 and strangely felt better in terms of energy, mood and ability to multitask while on the antibiotics. Unfortunately during this time, I repeatedly had my labs pulled and the titer never moved. Therefore, I made the difficult decision to have my tonsils removed in addition to nasal surgery. I had suffered repeatedly since the age of 12 a few times a year with sinus infections and Strep throat, so this didn't seem that far-fetched to me. The tonsils showed acute tonsillitis with lots of bacteria and debris but they "forgot" to culture the tonsils despite being repeatedly asked. Four weeks after the tonsillectomy, my lab work showed ASO went from 224 to 184 to 170 and DNase B went from 560 to 312 to 348. I re-pull labs each 12 months to monitor.

A year later he was better, yet still wouldn't have playdates with kids he noticed didn't wash their hands after they used the restroom, and he was scared of anyone that was sick or didn't feel well. Over time, we noticed certain things would set off his symptoms again, which always scares us. For instance, we tend to notice tics and loud behavior about 24-48 hours before a note comes home from school that Strep was found in his grade-level. (We have been very fortunate that the school works with us and shares any contagious illnesses when they happen).

Two years later, we found by introducing essential oils (particularly frankincense, oregano, cinnamon, clove, tea tree and copaiba) that he would not be susceptible to the usual triggers and his immune system could fight what would make others around him sick. We were also diligent with daily probiotics and vitamin D_3.

What types of practitioners did you find to be most helpful for your son's recovery?

We have been very fortunate to have found a psychologist familiar with long-term childhood illnesses that helped our family talk through the ups/downs and struggles. We had no idea how lonely that road would feel, and that person has been paramount in our family recovery.

While we are fortunate to have a good team of doctors around us, it is sad that for three years we were called by our old pediatrician and neurologist and told that our son had Tourette and he should be taken off antibiotics and Motrin and put on mind-altering medication. What they fail to understand is he doesn't have any symptoms when he is on Motrin and/or antibiotic use. If he truly had Tourette, the antibiotics and Motrin would have no effect. Although I must admit, if I hadn't seen this myself, I may never have believed it either. Sadly, we recently heard news that Child Protective Services had been called on a mother by someone that didn't believe in the treatment she was giving her child with PANDAS. There is a large community of parents that are going through this and are scared to address and talk about it for fear of backlash from the medical community. For anyone that says an infectious illness can't cause neurological issues, just ask a mother who feeds her child corn syrup or red dye... ask if her child acts different following eating this. I ask that we all take a step back and do what is right for our children's health and understand why an infectious illness may cause neuro-logical issues rather than debate if an infectious illness could cause neurological issues.

Do you have any helpful hints for other parents? Is there something you wish you knew early on in your son's healing journey?

There are certain supplements I wish I knew about earlier, includ-ing olive leaf extract, (especially as needed when a viral infection is present), QBC (a supplement containing quercetin, bromelain and vitamin C) and copaiba (an essential oil) as needed for inflamma-tion (as natural alternative to Motrin), daily vitamin D_3 for immune support, Daily Complete Omega, daily probiotic, daily methylfolate (different than folic acid) for his heterozygous MTHFR mutations 6 and 12, and PS (phosphatidylserine) as needed for sleep at night.

We had to make diet changes, and this is a crucial part to start early. We cut out gluten and restricted casein and sugar for two years, and now we have allowed casein back in his diet and mild amounts of gluten and sugar. This has been more work on me but has been good for our family as we cook more "whole food" dinners rather than grabbing something quick at a restaurant or grabbing something out of the pantry or freezer.

We now have our son using Listerine before brushing the teeth, then brushing teeth then using Listerine. We have all started this protocol and both illness and allergies are much less than without this protocol.

What are some of the most powerful healing tools you picked up on this journey?

In the last year and a half, unbelievably, the use of essential oils has brought our son back to 100%. Here is the protocol we used for the first 6-12 months:

We gave KidScents' MightyZyme chewable tablet twice a day, one to two ounces of Ningxia Juice twice a day. We performed an essential oil massage once a week and diffused three to four drops nightly of Thieves, thyme, frankincense and Peace and Calming, lavender and then Valor next. However, any of the oils can be diffused. We took the following essential oil capsules every day with a meal: three drops each of oregano, thyme, Thieves, frankincense, lavender and balsam fir or copaiba.

You can also apply these oils to the bottom of the feet. You may see a flare up of symptoms at first, which is a result of a detox reaction. The symptoms are always temporary. For maintenance we give him one capsule a day plus rubbing his feet at night with oils of oregano, cinnamon, clove, turmeric, frankincense and myrrh.

Sadly, we have followed the stories of many others that did not follow our path and instead went down the road of continued antibiotics, Advil and regular IVIG treatments that are better for short periods but not longer ones. Those families have not seen good results.

How is your son doing now?

He is doing great about five years later. He minimizes sugar and gluten and feels better for it. We did do family therapy as it really changed our family. The older sibling was largely ignored and developed germ fears after our overly careful measures at home. The therapy was helpful for him, and he is 100% well now.

What is the single most important thing you have learned from being on this healing journey with your child?

Life is precious. Organic, clean food with minimized sugar and gluten and daily supplements are an important part of giving your body the tools it needs to heal.

Maria's Story

"He came home one weekend afternoon from playing at a neighbor's house. He was enraged so much that he couldn't speak. He just slammed the front door, screaming and crying while he stomped upstairs, then slammed the door to his room so that the whole house shook. I thought, "If he's like this now, what's he going to be like as a teenager?" When he came downstairs a while later, I saw that he had ripped a massive clump of hair from his head, so much so that he looked a bit like a monk with a tonsure."

How would you describe your child before the onset of PANDAS/PANS/AE? What was she like?

My son was, for the most part, a very happy baby and toddler. In fact, he would do his "happy dance" because he felt so good and was so happy. He was always very sweet and generous.

Did your child have any of the "soft signs" of a pending chronic illness (such as allergies, chronic ear infections as a baby, eczema, dark circles under the eyes, attention issues, constipation, diarrhea, "tummy aches," etc.)?

My son had a tongue tie that prevented him from nursing well. He had trouble latching on when nursing and would alternately scream and cry because he wasn't getting enough, and he would nurse so forcefully that he would then projectile vomit.

He had severe colic as an infant and would arch his back when lying on his back. These were the days when doctors advised, "back to sleep," but my son had trouble sleeping while lying on his back because the colic was so painful. He was finally diagnosed with "silent reflux" at the age of 12 months after I persisted with his gastroenterologist, who performed an endoscopy on my son. My son developed a very painful diaper rash that was so acidic that it ate the skin off his bottom and led to a bloody diaper rash. His pediatrician recommended putting liquid Maalox or Mylanta on it because the alka-

linity of the minerals in these formulations balanced the acidity of his bowel movements. My son did not gain weight well and was put on a prescription of Pediasure. Although it helped somewhat with his weight gain, it didn't help with his acid reflux, so he was given a prescription of Prevacid.

When did you notice that something neurological was happening with your son? Were there any sudden changes that you noticed?

When he got to preschool when he was three years old, he had a lot of fun and made a lot of friends. Something happened, though, when he entered the fours (four year olds) program. When he was three, I was able to drop him off in the drop-off lane from my car. When he was four, however, he refused. I had to park my car in the parking lot and beg and plead for him to go to preschool as I walked him inside. Once inside, I had to stay for quite a while until he became comfortable enough for me to leave. By the time he reached kindergarten, his teacher related a few major meltdowns that he had had in the classroom. Because he got along so well with the other children in his class, I figured that these meltdowns were just hiccups in his transition to elementary school.

Even though he got along fantastically with other children, he never wanted to participate in after-school programs, sports or summer camps. At home, we never knew what his personality was going to be like: Dr. Jekyll or Mr. Hyde? It was like walking on eggshells around him. We never knew when he would get upset about the tiniest thing. I considered that he may have bipolar disorder, as my father, aunt and grandfather all had it.

The next big turning point was when he was in fourth grade. He came home one weekend afternoon from playing at a neighbor's house. He was enraged so much that he couldn't speak. He just slammed the front door, screaming and crying while he stomped upstairs, then slammed the door to his room so that the whole house shook. I thought, "If he's like this now, what's he going to be like as a teenager?" When he came downstairs a while later, I saw that he had ripped a massive clump of hair from his head, so much so that he looked a bit like a monk with a tonsure.

How was your child diagnosed? Did you experience any push-back from the doctors you sought out for help?

At this point, my husband and I realized that something was majorly wrong. I contacted the school psychologist at my son's school to have her be on the lookout for any issues at school. In the meantime, I had lunch with a friend of mine, who is a homotoxicologist, nutritionist and BioSET practitioner. My intention in having lunch with her was just to catch up and see how she was doing. I mentioned what had happened to my son, showed her the picture of what he had done to his hair, and she said to bring him in to see her as soon as possible, which I did the next week. I also made an appointment with our pediatrician for my son immediately.

Our pediatrician is one in a million, and she is the eighth or ninth pediatrician that we've had. I've cycled through a lot of them to find one that "gets it." She and I went through a list of possibilities that this episode could be due to: Lyme disease, PANDAS (chronic Strep), bipolar disorder and low iron. (Low iron, she said, is associated with trichotillomania, which is compulsive hair pulling). She ordered a blood test for Lyme looking at the different Lyme bands, as well as an Anti-Streptolysin O (ASO) test, which looks at the blood titer levels of Strep.

My pediatrician is also a fan of the Medical Medium, Anthony William, as am I, so she ordered blood tests looking at levels of Epstein-Barr virus, cytomegalovirus (CMV) and HHV-6, which are all troublesome herpetic viruses that he mentions in his book. Anthony William suggests, and many practitioners that I've spoken to agree, that Lyme disease itself is not the final issue. Instead, it is the underlying toxicity that attracts and retains viruses, especially herpetic viruses, to infect and retain residence in the body. These viruses lie dormant until times of stress. I can attest to this myself, as I have had shingles, which is also due to a herpetic virus, twice, and both times I was in states of extreme stress before its onset.

While we were waiting for my son's blood-test results, I took him to see my nutritionist friend. In her practice, she uses an electro-dermal screening device called a Zyto that reads electrical frequencies of organs, nutrients and pathogens in the body. Her Zyto screening of my son said that he had both a chronic Strep infection (PANDAS) as well as Lyme disease. It was a relief to know that there was an identifiable cause of my son's mood problems!

We got the blood test results the next week while we were on vacation in San Diego. His Anti-Streptolysin O titer level was extremely high at 1,204; the maximum high reference range is 1,205. In addition, his Lyme antibody count was at 266, well over the maximum reference-range level of 150. The Lyme Western blot test, which is controversial, showed that he was positive/reactive for nine IgG bands and one IgM band. The footnote in the blood test read, "As per CDC criteria, a Lyme disease IgG immunoblot test must show reactivity to at least five of 10 specific Borrelial proteins to be considered positive." While it was validating to see the blood-test results confirm what the Zyto machine found, I was angry at myself to think that he may have had these infections for years! As a health coach, I felt like I was supposed to know better!

Please tell me about your child's symptoms. How and when did these symptoms emerge? How did they affect your child? How did they affect your family?

My son had many classic symptoms of PANDAS and PANS, which includes Lyme disease. Most of all, he had severe mood swings, which I used to think were solely caused by low blood sugar. I used to call him "Mr. Mercurial Temperament" because I never knew when something, anything, would set him off into a violent rage. When he wasn't raging, he was the sweetest, kindest, most thoughtful and generous boy I'd ever met. He had a lot of somatic symptoms, such as headaches, stomach aches and problems sleeping. There were many days I kept him home from school because of his complaints of not feeling well. When I caught on that these symptoms usually appeared on a Monday, I realized he was avoiding school. He couldn't tell me why he didn't want to go to school, just that he hated it, even though he is a very bright child, does very well at school and has lots of friends at school. He would often tell me that he was depressed or sad, but he never knew why he felt that way. I thought it was highly unusual for a nine-year-old child to say that he's depressed. At some point, he developed a strange, throat-clearing cough that wasn't associated with any cold, allergies or sinus infection. He coughed this way so often that I wondered if this was a form of a tic or compulsion.

Did anything seem to "trigger" the first onset of your child's symptoms? Is there anything currently that you feel triggers the symptoms to come back?

Looking back, I see two major turning points in his PANS/PANDAS development. The first was when he was entering the fours program at preschool, and the second was after getting into a heated argument with some neighborhood children. Both of these point to stress being a trigger. Even though to me, these events may have seemed like no big deal, to him they were, and that's what matters.

What was the lowest point for you, your child, your family along this healing journey?

The low point for us was seeing the huge chunk of hair that my son pulled out from his head. To know that he was that frustrated and angry made me feel sad and worried.

What therapies did you try? What worked? What didn't work? Which therapies were the most helpful?

Because of my work as a health coach and as the media director and a board member of Epidemic Answers, I am very aware of the damage that antibiotics can do, so I chose to avoid them unless absolutely necessary. In addition, I am not a fan of removing parts of the body, such as in a tonsillectomy, as I believe that, given enough support, the body knows how to heal. I realize that they are the "standard of care" for most Western-medicine doctors, but I also know that children may have to be on them for years before results are seen. Our pediatrician agreed with treating my son herbally, nutritionally and homeopathically. We used antimicrobial herbal tinctures, colloidal silver, high-dose PharmaGABA and targeted homeopathics such as the DesBio Streptococcus series therapy. Other homeopathics that she suggested were for calming his stress and supporting his adrenals. She recommended, and I've heard other practitioners say this, that we treat the chronic Strep infection first, then the Lyme disease. I had already been giving my son GABA because I knew that it is calming and can help with anxiety and stress. However, we decided to quadruple the amount of GABA, and, to me, that made the biggest difference because it immediately eliminated the large majority of his angry episodes. We plan to start neurofeedback with Dr. Roseann Capanna-Hodge, an educational psychologist and neurofeedback practitioner who is also an Epidemic Answers board member if he shows stress-related symptoms in the future.

How is your son doing now? What do you do to support him in the aftermath of this experience?

My son is doing so much better now! I had already been giving him a strong foundation of nutrition and supplements, so these extra remedies were just added to the mix. Given that my son has been recovering from Sensory Processing Disorder (SPD) since the time that he was two, he has had the benefit of a cleaned-up diet, targeted supplements, visits to a naturopath and avoiding pharmaceuticals. I have done and continue to do what I can to make our home a haven for our boys. This includes earlier-than-typical bedtimes, lots of downtime and a non-toxic environment. We are not overscheduled, probably because both of my sons are not interested in playing sports. I have Himalayan salt lamps, essential oil diffusers, Stetzer dirty electricity filters and grounding pillowcases in each of their rooms, and I turn off the Wi-Fi router at night. In addition, there is no screen time after 6:00pm.

What is the single most important thing you have learned from being on this healing journey with your child?

I am constantly applying what I learn in one situation to myself, other family members, my clients and my public work. Given that my son benefitted from the recovery of my other son from Sensory Processing Disorder because my son was also mildly affected with it, I wondered if my other son also had PANS, Lyme or PANDAS. He didn't have major mood swings like my son did, but he was very clingy, even as a tween. We tested him, and sure enough, he also had PANDAS and Lyme. We are now treating him as well, but we had to clear Mycoplasma pneunomiae first for eight months before we could address Epstein-Barr virus, which will take another eight months or so. At some point after that, I'm assuming we'll address Strep and Lyme, but that may depend on what comes up as his highest priority in the Zyto scan. I found out that the younger children of two other moms who have recovered their older sons from autism and SPD also turned out to have PANDAS. We all found out our kids were diagnosed within a few months of each other, and we discovered this at the screening of "My Kid Is Not Crazy," a documentary about PANDAS. Our practitioners have told us that it's actually very typical for the younger sibling of a child with a neuro-developmental disorder to present with PANS/PANDAS. This is because the older child gets more of the toxic load from the mother and more effort is spent on the neurological aspects of these disorders. The older child may have PANS/PANDAS, but these immunological issues are dwarfed in comparison to autism, ADD/ADHD or SPD.

CHAPTER 3
HEALING PANS

Parents can easily get overwhelmed when a child has a condition like PANS — it's a lot to take in! The key is to take it one step at a time and start with the simple things that are within your control. In this chapter we have included an introduction to some healing fundamentals, and provided detailed information about therapies and approaches that can be helpful for children with PANS.

FIRST THINGS FIRST: THERE IS AN ORDER TO HEALING

There is no one way to heal, but there are foundational aspects that need to be addressed first when a child is suffering from a complex chronic illness. Chronic illness indicates that something (usually many things) are out of balance in the body. Although each person is individual and will have individual needs, there are some universal healing basics that need to be addressed before individualized and specific therapies will be effective.

EPIDEMIC ANSWERS' FOUR-STEP HEALING PLAN

Step One: Take Away the Bad Stuff and Add Back in the Good Stuff

Before beginning any individualized healing approach, it is important to remove as many stressors to the body as possible and give the body what it needs to heal.

Take away the bad stuff. Anything you can do to green your home and eliminate exposures to environmental toxins or stressors is going to help your child heal.

Use the following checklist to see if you have thought about the many ways to reduce your child's "total load" by keeping a "green" and safe home. You don't have to do these all today—consider this a list to work through over time.

◆ Avoid bringing new furnishings and building materials such as new carpets, paints, glues, linoleum, insulation, siding and cabinets, etc., into your home.

◆ Have you reduced exposure to electromagnetic radiation in your home? Ways to reduce exposure:

- Get rid of WiFi (Hardwire your home for internet instead—a lot of families who have recovered from PANS do this).

- If you can't get rid of WiFi, at least turn it off at night and make sure your child's bed is not near a WiFi router, SmartMeter or 5G antenna.

- Have your child use any electronic devices (smartphones, tablets, etc.) in airplane mode, and only use a hardwired device to search the internet.

- Do not let your child use a cell phone.

- Use *corded* phones instead of cordless phones.

- If your home has a SmartMeter, see if you can get rid of it or talk to an expert who can do SmartMeter shielding. SmartMeters are a significant source of harmful electromagnetic radiation.

- Do not let your child have a fan, dehumidifier, alarm clock or other electronic appliance near his/her bed while sleeping.

- Move your child's bed away from any large electronic appliances such as refrigerators, TVs, computers, WiFi routers, induction ovens, etc. (Even if the child's bed is on the other side of a wall, there is exposure).

♦ Have you checked your child's toys to ensure they are non-toxic? Beware of cheap costume jewelry that may contain heavy metals such as cadmium and lead, cheaply manufactured plastics or anything containing vinyl (beach balls, rubber duckies, etc.).

♦ Have you checked for mold in the walls of your home, bathrooms and kitchen? If you can smell mold or see mold anywhere in your home, this could be a real problem for your child. Consider mold remediation.

♦ Has your home been checked for radon gas? Radon in the water?

♦ Were your walls painted with conventional VOC (Volatile Organic Compounds) paint (most paint brands) or did you use "green" non-VOC paint?

♦ Was your home built before 1974? Lead paint can be present in homes built before this date.

♦ Does your hand soap or toothpaste contain triclosan? (Read the label.) If so, choose a safer brand. Triclosan negatively impacts the endocrine and immune systems.

♦ Have you changed your laundry soap, fabric softener and dryer sheets to non-toxic products without fragrances? You can just skip the dryer sheets all together—they are a significant source of toxin exposure.

♦ Have you changed your cleaning products to natural cleaning products that don't have chemicals? Use non-toxic cleaning products such as baking soda, vinegar, lemon, tea tree oil, thyme oil and/or organic products to clean.

♦ Do you use disinfectants in your home? Swap them out for disinfectants that contain natural ingredients like vinegar, thyme and other essential oils.

♦ Do you use bleach? Best to skip the bleach all together.

◆ Are you using natural pest-control products in your house and attic? Many people prefer using more natural products that contain essential oils.

◆ Is the wood in and around your home pressure-treated? This includes playground equipment. Many of these wood products contain arsenic and/or formaldehyde.

◆ Do you cook, microwave or store food in plastic? Consider using glass, stainless steel or cast iron for cooking and storing food. If you do need to use plastic, avoid #3, #6 & #7 plastic products (look on the bottom of the bottle/container) as they can contain harmful chemicals.

◆ Have you checked to make sure you are not cooking with aluminum pots, non-stick pans (such as those containing Teflon) or any other chemically laden cooking utensils or pots?

◆ Do you have a good indoor air filter?

◆ Have you removed the compact fluorescent light bulbs and replaced them with incandescent bulbs? CFLs contain mercury. If you break one, the EPA recommends that you follow a complex and detailed clean up protocol (including evacuating pets and people from the area) because the materials in the bulb are so hazardous.

◆ Have you installed a good quality water filter to eliminate chemicals like chlorine, fluoride and other toxins found in municipal/town water?

◆ Have you removed perfumed candles and other chemically laden perfumed soap products from your home?

◆ Do you or anyone in your home use perfume or cologne? Perfumes and colognes contain endocrine disrupting chemicals.

◆ Do you have a conventional mattress or an organic/natural mattress? Conventional mattresses contain flame retardants and other chemicals.

◆ Have you replaced your vinyl shower curtains and liners to cotton or linen ones?

◆ Do you use a microwave? Instead, consider using a steam oven or small infrared convection oven or toaster oven for the countertop for fast and easy reheating and cooking.

◆ Is your child exposed to tobacco smoke? Eliminate tobacco exposure whenever possible. Second-hand smoke is dangerous for everyone.

◆ Are your child's clothes made from organic materials? Choose organic cotton materials for clothing when possible. If you do buy new clothes, be sure to wash them several times before wearing them to remove chemicals.

◆ Have you removed your wall-to-wall carpets? These unfortunately contain many toxin exposures.

◆ Do you avoid pharmaceutical medications for acute illnesses unless absolutely necessary? Consult with your integrative healthcare practitioner to determine the best way to manage acute illnesses for your child. Because most pharmaceutical medications are chemicals that have been altered to be different from something in nature (in order to be "patentable"), your body recognizes the compounds as foreign—this is why many pharmaceutical medications have side effects. It's your body's way of telling you that it is dealing with something unknown and toxic.

◆ Do you routinely open the windows in your home to let in fresh air? Indoor air contains far more pollutants than outdoor air, so let the outside in!

◆ Does your child wear sunscreen 24-7? Many sunscreens contain toxic ingredients. Despite what you may have been told about sun exposure, it may not be such a good idea to totally block the sun. It is important to remember that wearing sunscreen prevents your child from receiving the benefits of natural sunlight, including the production of vitamin D that occurs when the sunlight hits your skin. Let your child get a responsible amount of sunlight on his/her skin to encourage healthy vitamin D levels. Moderate sun exposure (especially first thing in the morning) is important to regulate circadian rhythms (for proper sleep) and healthy immune function. If your child does wear sunscreen, be sure to check databases of safe sunscreens available at MadeSafe.org or EWG.org.

◆ Does your child have consistent and early bedtimes? Remember, nighttime is when our bodies detoxify, and they can't get rid of all of the toxins listed above if they aren't sleeping. If your child is having trouble sleeping, make sure they are exposed to natural sunlight during the day, and don't use any devices for two hours before bedtime.

For more information about products that may be harmful to your child's body see www.epidemicanswers.org, www.ewg.org, and www.madesafe.org.

Add back in the good stuff. While removing stressors from your child's life, it is equally important to simultaneously support your child's body with all the things that a healthy body needs to thrive. Food is a great place to start. Clean, nourishing food is foundational to healing. The other "good stuff" to add back may include natural sunlight, clean water, natural exposures (such as forests and beaches), movement/exercise and sleep.

Let's start by looking at food as a health support. There is much controversy around what constitutes a healthy diet. In 2009, Michael Pollan wrote a book titled *Food Rules*, which tried to provide some simplified guidelines about how to eat healthy in a world replete with conflicting information about diet. But even that book was overtaken by yet another book by Frank Lipman, MD titled *The New Food Rules*, which identified some flaws in Pollan's thinking. And this is just the tip of the food and diet iceberg. It's a contentious subject with a seemingly endless number of opinions. So what is a parent to do? What should you feed a child with PANS?

Why not start with following in the footsteps of those families who have successfully reversed chronic inflammatory conditions (like PANS, autism, asthma, ADHD) in their own children? Most integrative practitioners who treat children with PANS and many families who have recovered their children will agree on the following basic "food rules," for an optimal diet for sick kids:

- Eat whole foods
- Eliminate all processed foods (anything that comes in a package/box)
- Eliminate sugar
- Eat a wide variety of foods (heavy on the vegetables)
- Eat clean protein
- Eat good fats
- Hydrate adequately with clean water

Want to dive deeper into the details? Every child has different nutritional needs, so please remember that there is no perfect diet for everyone. Different medical conditions have different nutritional needs, so consider working with an integrative nutrition professional to help tailor a diet to your child's particular nutritional needs. As we have learned over the years talking to doctors, nutritionists/dietitians and families who have recovered their children from all varieties of chronic health conditions (including PANS), there are certain nutritional strategies and approaches that are excellent for supporting the healing process. We've created a checklist for you to consider as you design a tailored diet for your child's needs.

- Is your family eating a whole-foods diet?
- Have you removed all fast foods and processed foods?
- Are you buying organic food whenever possible?
- Have you removed GMOs (genetically modified foods) from your diet? Seventy percent of processed foods contain

GMOs. The most common source of GMOs are soy, canola, corn and sugar beets. Always buy those foods organically, if you buy them at all.

- ◆ Are you limiting the following foods in your child's diet?
  - • Sugars (including soft drinks, teas, juices, sports drinks, etc.)
  - • Refined carbohydrates
  - • Hydrogenated oils, vegetable oils like corn oil, soy oil or canola oil?

- ◆ Have you done a food allergy and food sensitivity test for your child? Undetected food sensitivities can wreak havoc on a body trying to combat a condition like PANS. Many conventionally trained physicians do not yet accept food sensitivities as clinically meaningful or relevant to health and wellness. Conversely, most holistic and integrative practitioners know that food sensitivities are often directly related to any number of chronic symptoms, including eczema, bedwetting, mood and behavior disorders, developmental delays, and many, many others. Countless parents have found that removing trigger foods (not necessarily forever!) from their children's diets can profoundly impact the intensity and frequency of symptoms. Most parents are not even aware that their children have these hidden food sensitivities—they are a hugely underrecognized problem. For more information, see Doris Rapp, MD's books *Is This Your Child?* and *Is This Your Child's World?*

- ◆ See the Epidemic Answers website for more information about food sensitivity testing: https://epidemicanswers.org/reference-library/allergies-and-sensitivities/allergy-sensitivity-testing/

- ◆ Have you eliminated any possible trigger foods from your child's diet? Some of the most common food sensitivities include:

- Gluten/wheat (often includes oats due to cross-contamination)
- Casein/dairy
- Corn
- Sugar
- Eggs
- Soy
- Nuts
- Citrus
- Phenols
- Artificial colors
- Artificial flavors
- Natural flavors
- Salicylates
- Chemical preservatives

◆ Is your child getting protein for breakfast before going to school?

◆ Is your child getting healthy snacks for school?

◆ Are you using salt with minerals such as Himalayan salts, Celtic sea salt, or RealSalt?

◆ Is your child drinking enough filtered water?

◆ Are you including enough good-quality fats in your child's diet? Sources of good fats include:

- Coconut oil
- Olive oil
- Avocados
- Nuts
- Wild salmon
- Small wild fish like mackerel, sardines, etc.

- Organic, pastured chicken, turkey, duck, goose

- Organic, pastured ghee

- Organic, pasture-raised eggs

- Organic, pastured beef, lamb, bison

- Essential fatty acids from: cod liver oil, hemp seeds, flax seeds, evening primrose oil, borage oil, walnut oil

◆ Is your child getting raw fermented foods daily in their diet? Raw fermented foods may include raw pickles, kimchi, sauerkraut, yogurt, kefir and more. See Sandor Katz's book *Wild Fermentation* or Donna Gates' *Body Ecology Diet* for more information about the importance of eating fermented foods. They help rebuild a damaged microbiome.

◆ Have you checked the Environmental Working Group website (www.ewg.org) for information about which fruits and vegetables have the most pesticides? See their list the "Dirty Dozen" to discover which foods to buy organic and the "Clean Fifteen" to discover which fruits and vegetables contain the least amount of pesticides.

◆ Are you finding creative ways to get your child to eat leafy greens and vegetables? Children should eat 9 to 11 servings of fruits and vegetables (heavy on the vegetables) per day.

Changes to diet do not have to happen overnight. Use the above list as a series of goals that you work towards, and do the best you can with what you've got.

While you are working on diet changes, there are many ways to **add back in the *other* good stuff** to your child's daily life. Following is a basic checklist of lifestyle factors for you to consult:

◆ Is your getting enough rest at night? If your child has trouble falling asleep, limit exposures to devices containing blue lights (smartphones, tablets, computers, TVs) several hours before bedtime because blue lights suppress the production of melatonin, an important hormone required for sleep.

Also remember to set early bedtimes—even earlier than you think is "normal."

◆ Did your child get outside today? Exposure to outdoor environments is critical to health.

◆ Did your child see the sun today? Without sunscreen or sunglasses?

◆ Did your child touch the earth or a tree today? Research is now proving what many have long known to be true... touching the earth, or trees or other natural elements connected to the earth, has positive health benefits, including lowering cortisol levels, reducing inflammation and speeding healing.

◆ Has your child had time to unwind, decompress, be still, or reflect today?

The checklists above include things you can mostly do on your own. If you need help, there are people out there who love working with families striving to make healthy lifestyle changes. And this brings us to Step Two!

Step Two: Get Help

You can't be expected to know all the things in your home that might be negatively impacting your child's health, nor are you expected to have a graduate degree in nutrition! That is why it is important to know that there are many health and wellness professionals that can help you up the learning curve.

Talk to a Certified Health Coach

A health coach is someone who can help a family navigate the healing journey. They can:

◆ Support a family as they make diet and lifestyle changes

◆ Help identify underlying root causes

◆ Help identify toxic stressors in a child's life

- ◆ Recommend health care providers who fit your child's unique needs

Epidemic Answers hosts a directory of health coaches and offers a free consult with a health coach as a way to get you started. To connect with a health coach visit: https://epidemicanswers.org/free-health-coach-consultation/

Find an Integrative or Functional Medicine Practitioner

Most physicians were trained to manage the symptoms of chronic illnesses, rather than treat the underlying causes. There is a better way. Work with a practitioner experienced in treating the whole body and reversing chronic illness. Visit the Epidemic Answers Practitioner Directory at https://epidemicanswers.org/practitioners/practitioner/ to find an integrative practitioner in your area. Often times, practitioners will find that affected children have:

- ◆ Intestinal dysbiosis, an imbalance in intestinal bacteria and microbes (not enough good germs and too many bad germs)

- ◆ Nutritional deficiencies (such as low magnesium, iron, zinc, or essential fatty acids), even if they have a good diet

- ◆ Evidence of oxidative stress (too many free radicals causing damage to cells and tissues)

- ◆ Structural, sensory or other physiological abnormalities

And remember to ask other parents in your community who have found practitioners that they love. You are looking for a practitioner who believes in identifying root causes and does not believe in suppressing symptoms with medications. Ask around!

Some types of practitioners who are more experienced in this approach include:

- ◆ Integrative physicians

- ◆ Holistic physicians

- ◆ Osteopathic physicians

- ◆ Naturopathic physicians

- ◆ Chiropractic physicians

- ◆ Homeopaths

- ◆ Holistic or integrative nurse practitioners or physician assistants

Find a Support Group

There are numerous organizations set up to assist families with a multitude of healing issues. Nearly all of the topics covered on this book – from eating whole foods to methylation issues – have support groups. The PANDAS Network hosts support groups that you can find online: http://www.pandasnetwork.org/supportgroups/

The New England PANS/PANDAS Association also hosts support groups and also provides a treasure trove of information on PANS. We highly recommend a site visit:

http://www.nepans.org/support-groups.html

It's okay to ask for help. No one should walk this path alone.

Step Three: Rebalance the Imbalances

Once you've established a good foundation for healing through diet and lifestyle modifications, it is important to try to identify and address any existing imbalances in the body. Some common ongoing imbalances commonly seen in children with PANS include:

- ◆ **Gut Dysbiosis.** Living in your gut are trillions of bacteria and other microorganisms that are essential to the most basic biological mechanisms required for human life such as digestion, energy production, immune function and detoxification. Gut dysbiosis means that there is an upset in the natural balance of microorganisms in your gut. When your gut is dysbiotic, this means that the "bad germs" (or opportunistic germs) begin to edge out the "good germs." When the bad germs edge out the good germs, basic biological processes begin to breakdown, and symptoms (like diarrhea or constipation) begin to appear. Not all symptoms of gut dysbiosis are obvious. Because gut dysbiosis can lead to any number of physiological problems throughout the body, it can be responsible for symptoms as varied as depression and breathing difficulties. When a body is unable to effectively combat the bad germs in the gut (or elsewhere in the body) a state of immune dysregulation can occur. This is of critical importance in children with PANS as imbalances in the gut microbiome are directly associated with the development of autoimmunity. Many people with autoimmune diseases—including PANS—have been able to fully reverse their conditions by addressing gut dysbiosis, and restoring natural balance to the germs in their guts.

◆ **Nutritional Deficiencies.** A corollary of gut dysbiosis is that it can cause nutritional deficiencies. Although it is not the only cause of nutritional deficiencies (nutrient-depleted food, limited diversity of foods, Standard American Diet, etc., are all causes), it can exacerbate nutritional imbalances. Gut bacteria play a critical role in breaking down, synthesizing and processing our food so that we can utilize the nutrients within. For example, some helpful gut bacteria actually make B vitamins as a byproduct. We use these B vitamins for everything from energy production to immune function. If we do not have these bacteria in our guts, we may be deficient in B vitamins. Some nutritional deficiencies can be easily addressed through eating a healthy and diverse diet of nutrient-dense, whole foods.

Some find nutrient testing helpful. There are a variety of ways to test for nutrient status. Some involve blood or urine tests, and others can be done using hands-on approaches such as applied kinesiology. Ask your healthcare practitioner to test for nutritional deficiencies in your child. Common nutrient deficiencies seen in children with PANS include:

- Vitamin D
- B vitamins, especially niacin and B_{12}
- Vitamin C

- Essential fatty acids
- Zinc
- Magnesium
- Selenium
- Iodine
- Iron
- Trace minerals
- And more

Step Four: Rehabilitation and Reintegration

There are many techniques used to enhance function in the body. These techniques won't be as effective if the underlying imbalances (already discussed) have not been addressed first. For example, a child with significant nutritional deficiencies won't get as much benefit from brain stimulation exercises to improve focus until this imbalance has been addressed. Once the basic imbalances have been addressed, there are many techniques to rewire or rehabilitate the brain, and reintegrate the brain and body to optimize function. Following are just a few examples of functions that often need to be reintegrated, restored, or rehabilitated in children with symptoms of PANS:

- ◆ **Retained Primitive Reflexes.** Primitive reflexes emerge as early as nine weeks *in utero* and are fully present at birth. Primitive reflexes are automatic movements, executed without thinking. They assist in the birthing process, are essential for the infant's survival in the first months of life, and provide training for many later skills. Primitive reflexes are considered "aberrant," however, if they remain active beyond age 6–12 months. They are supposed to be "integrated" by this age, which means that the brain should inhibit them from happening. However, many children who have developmental or inflammatory conditions never fully integrated some of these reflexes.

The continued presence of any of twelve primitive and postural reflexes is a sign of central nervous system (CNS) immaturity, which can have a profound impact upon a child's development, learning, behavior and even immune function. To see if your child has retained reflexes, see an occupational therapist, developmental physician, developmental optometrist, neuromovement or neurodevelopmental practitioner trained in this field. Some helpful websites include:

- www.masgutovamethod.com

- www.anatbanielmethod.com

- www.blombergrmt.com

- www.moveplaythrive.com

◆ **Vision.** Vision is an often overlooked function in the body because it is commonly confused with eyesight. Eyesight is the same as visual acuity: how clear something is. Glasses can correct eyesight. Vision is an interaction between the eyes and the brain. It is the learned ability to focus on and give meaning to what is seen. Many children have good eyesight, but poor vision, and this can impact learning, movement, behavior and more. To improve vision, parents can seek help from a developmental optometrist, who can prescribe vision therapy to rehabilitate the entire visual system, if it was at any point impeded by neuroinflammation or arrested development. Too often, parents just assume that particular behaviors or symptoms their child displays are related to their child's diagnosis, when in fact they are developmental vision problems or visual dysfunction that can be addressed through therapies. Think of vision therapy as neurological training or rehabilitation for the entire visual system: eyes, brain and body. It can be a game-changer for many children.

One of the key goals of this therapy is to have children process information with both eyes simultaneously. When the left and right hemispheres in the brain are working together more efficiently, then so do the eyes! Simple tasks such as throwing and catching a ball or putting pegs in holes on a board or throwing bean bags at a target can now be accomplished. More sophisticated functions such as visual-motor skills (writing, reading), organizational skills, the ability to process language and gain visual thinking skills will all develop gradually.

- **Hearing,** like vision, is an often overlooked sensory function that can be impacted as a result of neuroinflammation. Children with PANS may benefit from listening therapy (like Tomatis therapy) or Auditory Integration Therapy (AIT) or Sound Stimulation, all of which are types of auditory therapy that can retrain the brain to help normalize hearing, senses and brain processing. These approaches can help improve: auditory processing, sensory processing, speech, language, focus, concentration, balance, coordination and more.

I'M FOLLOWING THE FOUR-STEP PLAN, NOW WHAT?

Many times when parents embark on the healing journey with their children, they feel like they've done *everything* and still their child is not getting better. Sometimes it helps to have a "brainstorm" list—a list of questions for you to consider to see what else might be helpful for your child. What stones are unturned? We've compiled a list of questions that come from parents who have "been there" and "done that." Maybe there is a useful pearl of wisdom for your child with PANS in this checklist?

- Have you confirmed that there are auto-antibodies through a Cunningham Panel?

- Has your child been tested for possible food sensitivities and allergies? Including gluten/wheat and casein/dairy?

- Have you checked for nutritional deficiencies? Genova Diagnostics is a diagnostic laboratory company that has a test called the NutrEval that looks for:
  - Malabsorption
  - Dysbiosis
  - Cellular energy
  - Mitochondrial metabolism
  - Neurotransmitter metabolism
  - Vitamin deficiencies
  - Toxin exposure
  - Detoxification need

- Have you identified any bacteria or yeast overgrowth in your child's gut? There are now many companies that allow you to send in a sample of stool to be tested for microbial imbalances. Consider the following testing companies: uBiome, Viome, Genova, Doctors Data or Great Plain Laboratories.

- Have you checked for neurotransmitter imbalances? Neurorelief (Neurosciences Laboratory) is a specialty lab that tests neurotransmitters to determine chemical imbalances in the brain.

- Have you considered working with a homeopath to help manage symptoms like anxiety or OCD? Remedies commonly used for anxiety include:
  - *Aconite*
  - *Chamomila*
  - *Gervanius*

- Many homeopaths can also talk to you about Bach flower essences which can be helpful for anxiety, worry, fear or other emotional symptoms.

- ◆ Have you considered using essential oils both as antimicrobials to combat infections and for therapeutic purposes? Some favorites to ask your practitioner about include:
  - **Vetiver** for anxiety for its calming properties and for reducing inflammation
  - **Frankincense** is anti-inflammatory and is used for focus, immune stimulation, and it is also antibacterial and antiviral
  - **Sandalwood** for focus, memory, calming, and for its antiviral and antibacterial properties
  - **Cedarwood** for focus, and its antibacterial, antifungal, anti-inflammatory properties
  - **Oregano** for antimicrobial properties
  - **Lavender** for its anti-anxiety and calming properties
  - **Thyme** for its antimicrobial properties
  - **Thieves oil** (a combination of oils) for its antimicrobial properties
  - **Tea tree oil** for its antifungal properties
- ◆ Have you considered working with a homeopath or homotoxicologist to help the body drain and detoxify?
- ◆ Have you considered working with a homeopath to create nosodes (specific remedies made from the pathogens affecting your child) to combat stubborn infections such as:
  - *Mycoplasma*
  - Epstein-Barr virus
  - *Streptococcus*
  - *Bartonella*
  - *Borrelia*
  - *Babesia*

- Have you considered adding in a probiotic supplement (or fermented food) into your child's daily routine? Some ideas for probiotic support include:
  - Kefir, yogurts, fermented vegetables, umeboshi plums
  - Bravo yogurt
  - Some probiotic supplements to ask your practitioner about include: VSL#3, Gut Pro, Dr. Ohirra's Live Cultured Probiotics, Garden of Life, Klaire Labs
- Have you talked to your practitioner about using herbs, essential oils and other natural supplements to address infections? Some helpful antimicrobial herbs and supplements to ask about include:
  - Berberine
  - Olive leaf
  - Oil of oregano
  - Grapefruit seed extract
  - Propolis
  - Biocidin
  - Banderol
  - Garlic
  - Samento (cat's claw)
  - Quina
  - Stevia
  - Argentyn or Smart Silver colloidal silver
  - Apple cider vinegar for gargling
  - Manuka honey
- Have you talked to your practitioner about supplements that can reduce the damage from chronic inflammation? Some powerful supplements include:
  - Turmeric/curcumin

- N-acetylcysteine (NAC)

- Vitamin C (ascorbic acid)

- Medicinal mushrooms such as reishi, cordyceps and more

◆ Have you considered using regular epsom salts baths to help your child detoxify?

◆ Have you talked to your practitioner about using digestive aids to facilitate digestion and extraction of nutrients from food:

  - Betaine hydrochloric acid

  - Digestive enzymes with DPP-IV for gluten and casein intolerances

  - Proteolytic enzymes

  - BiCarb

  - Bromelain

  - Papaya

◆ Have you looked for ways to help lower your and your child's stress levels? Viruses, bacteria and other pathogens become more active when the body is in a state of stress. Some ideas include:

  - Teaching your child ways to self-regulate with practices such as prayer, meditation, yoga, qi gong, tai chi and the Emotional Freedom Technique (tapping).

  - Techniques such as EMDR (Eye Movement Desensitization Retraining) and jin shin jyutsu can lower stress levels for your child, as well. These are done with a trained practitioner.

OTHER IMPORTANT THERAPIES AND APPROACHES

There are literally hundreds of important and effective therapies and modalities that can be used to help support your child's healing process. At the end of this book we have provided a glossary that includes definitions of various healing modalities that can benefit a child with PANS. Again, a bio-individual approach must be taken, and only you and your integrative health care practitioner can decide which therapies are best for your child. We have included a few of these therapies in the next section which addresses the psychological impact of PANS on the child and family, but there are many more approaches that are worth learning about. Please see the glossary to learn more about some of these approaches.

THE PSYCHOLOGICAL IMPACT OF PANS ON THE CHILD AND THE FAMILY

A chronic medical illness in childhood often causes an increase in psychological difficulties. And, in the case of children with PANS, these problems are compounded because the nature of the illness itself creates so many unique psychological symptoms.

A child with PANS can exhibit signs of anxiety, obsessive compulsive thoughts and behavior (OCD), rage and anger, behavioral dysregulation, anorexia, increased depression and even thoughts of suicide. It is especially important to address the psychological component as well as the biomedical component for the best possible outcome.

Several types of licensed mental health professionals work with children in psychological distress. Psychologists, social workers, counselors and specialists with advanced degrees have a variety of credentials and training. Finding the right one for you requires patience.

Psychotherapy or counseling refer to a range of treatments that can help with mental-health issues, emotional problems, and behavioral symptoms like those seen in PANS. This type of support empowers clients to identify, understand and change troubling emotions, thoughts and behavior.

Psychotherapy and counseling can help children understand and resolve problems, challenge negative self-talk and beliefs, and help to modify behavior. Also, children receiving treatment often learn to cope with intense emotions more effectively. Holistically minded clinicians will also incorporate spirituality, energy work, bodywork and other healing modalities into sessions as well.

THE IMPORTANCE OF PSYCHOLOGICAL SUPPORT FOR THE ENTIRE FAMILY

PANS is not just a child's medical matter. It's a family matter, too. The behaviors and mood of a child affected with this neuropsychiatric disorder affect the whole emotional atmosphere of the family. It often derails a family's dynamics, causes conflicts between siblings and creates a tremendous amount of stress on the marital relationship. Even after treatment, the children and the family often have Post-Traumatic Stress Disorder (PTSD). Thus, it is crucial that the proper psychotherapy is in place to assist all members of the family to help bring homeostasis back to the family system.

DIFFERENT TYPES OF PSYCHOTHERAPY MODALITIES

Therapists use a variety of tools and techniques to support a child's body and brain, as well as help the entire family. The body is designed to deal with stress first. Therefore, incorporating stress-reduction therapies is essential to the healing process.

There are differences between traditional psychotherapy and integrative body-mind psychotherapy. Traditional psychotherapy works with the conscious mind using conventional talk therapy methods and provides techniques to alleviate particular complaints and symptoms with the conscious control of the mind. In other words, clients are taught to access their rational mind centers.

Integrative body-mind psychotherapy differs from traditional psychotherapy in that it operates on the premise that the subconscious is really in control and that the body is part of that subconscious mind structure. When the body holds stress, it can impact both brain and body. The body holds physical stress (e.g., headaches, chronic pain, etc.), so working to release that tension through a variety of techniques and therapies is integral to treatment. Further, energy psychotherapy or energy medicine refers to the integration of energy work practices such as body tapping (EFT), holding, visualization, spirituality, systemic or family constellations and reiki into the practice of psychotherapy.

Tools and techniques that can support a child with PANS include:

- Psychotherapy
- CBT (Cognitive Behavioral Therapy)
- DBT (Dialectical Behavior Therapy)
- EMDR (Eye Movement Desensitization and Reprocessing)
- EFT/tapping (Emotional Freedom Technique)
- ERP (Exposure Therapy)
- Hypnosis
- Neurofeedback
- Biofeedback
- PEMF/BRT (Pulsed Electromagnetic Field Therapy/Bioregulation Therapy)
- Energy work

PSYCHOTHERAPY

In psychotherapy, therapists and psychologists apply scientifically validated techniques to help people develop healthier, more effective habits. It is a process; therapists treat psychological problems through communication and relationship development between an individual and a trained mental health professional. There are many approaches to psychotherapy, including cognitive-behavioral (CBT), behavior therapy, exposure therapy (ERP) and more. The goal of psychotherapy is to help individuals work through their problems in healthy ways. Through the psychotherapy process, one learns how to take control of their life and respond to challenging situations with healthy coping skills.

CBT

Cognitive Behavioral Therapy (CBT) is a type of psychotherapy that works on changing one's thoughts and ultimately behaviors. The goal of CBT is to change our thought patterns or beliefs (distorted or valid), attitudes, and ultimately our behavior to help us face our challenges and more effectively work toward our goals.

ERP

A type of Cognitive Behavioral Therapy is Exposure Therapy. Exposure Response and Prevention Therapy (ERP) is used with children and individuals who have obsessions and compulsions or Obsessive-Compulsive Disorder. Essentially with ERP, the person is exposed to their trigger and learns how to be uncomfortable to the point where they can ignore their trigger. Over time, through exposure, psychoeducation, and cognitive behavioral therapy, the person learns to respond differently to these triggers, leading to a decrease in the frequency of compulsions and the intensity of obsessions.

DBT

Dialectical Behavioral Therapy (DBT) is a type of psychotherapy that combines cognitive and behavioral therapies. The goal of DBT is to identify and change negative thinking patterns and destructive behaviors into positive outcomes. DBT skills include skills for mindfulness, emotion regulation, distress tolerance, and interpersonal effectiveness.

EMDR

Eye Movement Desensitization and Reprocessing, or EMDR, is a powerful psychotherapy technique originated by Francine Shapiro, PhD. It is very successful in helping people who suffer from trauma, anxiety, panic, disturbing memories, post-traumatic stress and many other emotional problems. Tactile, audio and visual stimulation is used to activate the opposite sides of the brain to help release emotional experiences that are "trapped" in the nervous system. "Whatever fires together wires together." Therefore, the goal is to reprocess the trauma and allow the "rational brain" to kick in to free the "emotional brain" of the high levels of emotion tied to the trauma to achieve a more peaceful state.

EFT/Tapping - Emotional Freedom Technique

EFT (also known as tapping) is a tool used for physical, emotional and performance issues. EFT operates on the premise that no matter what part of your life needs improvement, there are unresolved issues in the way. Any emotional stress can impede the human body's ability to heal itself. EFT works like emotional acupressure to quickly, gently and easily release negative emotions and beliefs that are at the root of the problem. EFT is a form of psychological acupressure, based on the same energy meridians used in traditional acupuncture to treat physical and emotional ailments for over five thousand years. Simple tapping with the fingertips is used to input kinetic energy onto specific meridians on the head and chest while you think about your particular problem and make statements.

Hypnosis

Hypnotherapy involves the induction of a trance-like condition, where the patient is actually in an enhanced state of awareness, concentrating entirely on the therapist's voice. In this state, the therapist calms the client using progressive-relaxation techniques to help suppress the conscious mind, allowing the subconscious mind to become more open. The therapist then suggests ideas, concepts and lifestyle adaptations to the patient, the seeds of which become firmly planted for positive change. Hypnotherapy aims to reprogram patterns of thoughts, behavior, and negative core beliefs within the mind, helping to eliminate irrational fears, phobias, negative thoughts and suppressed emotions.

NEUROFEEDBACK

Neurofeedback treats a variety of conditions in a safe and effective manner because it works at the subconscious level. It creates changes in the brain by creating new electrical activity through a process of measurement and reinforcement with the use of computers. Quite simply, brainwaves start changing at a subconscious level through reinforcement with the use of computers. The brain learns to self-regulate, which calms the nervous system, reducing or eliminating symptoms.

BIOFEEDBACK

Biofeedback is a technique that helps the client learn how to control heart rate, skin temperature and breath. When one has a chronic illness, learning how to self-regulate one's bodily functions can bring pain- and stress-relief by balancing the parasympathetic and sympathetic nervous system.

With biofeedback, one is connected to electrical sensors that measure and give information (feedback) about the body (bio). This feedback helps one focus on making subtle changes in the body, such as relaxing certain muscles, to achieve the desired results, such as reducing pain or controlling body temperature to reduce stress. It differs from neurofeedback because it requires conscious control over one's thoughts and autonomic functions. Biofeedback gives one the power to use thoughts to control the body, often reducing stress or improving a health condition or physical performance.

PEMF/BRT

PEMF is an acronym for Pulsed Electromagnetic Field therapy. PEMF is a type of therapy that promotes cellular communication, which in turn enhances self-healing and wellness. PEMF is a way to alter a body's energy fields to improve cellular functioning. Controlled and pulsed electromagnetic frequencies (PEMF) can deliver health enhancing EMFs to the cells.

BIOREGULATION THERAPY (BRT)

This is a unique approach to health and wellness that uses Bio-feedback and PEMF-based electromagnetic technology to help the body better self-regulate, adapt, and heal naturally. It helps to align with the body so the brain can work better.

ENERGY/BODY WORK

REIKI

One form of energy therapy is reiki, which is a Japanese technique for stress reduction and relaxation that also promotes healing. It is a specific form of energy healing, in which hands are placed just off the body or lightly touching the body, as in "laying on of hands." In a reiki session, the practitioner is seeking to transmit universal life energy to the client.

This unseen "life force energy" flows through all of us. If one's "life force energy" is low, then we are more likely to get sick or feel stress. When our life energy is at the optimal level, it helps promote happiness and healthiness within the body. This therapy deepens relaxation and initiates healing. It can also reduce pain and decrease other symptoms you may be experiencing.

CRANIOSACRAL THERAPY

Another effective bodywork/energy healing modality is craniosacral therapy. On a physical level, this therapy offers gentle manipulation of the cranium and the body to relieve pain and tension in the body by helping to regulate the flow of cerebrospinal fluid. On a deeper level, craniosacral therapists are trained to work with clients in a trance-like state, allowing the client to release emotional trauma from the body and the mind. Clients often report a feeling of deep relaxation thought to be caused by an increase of endorphins.

CHAPTER 4
ASK THE EXPERTS

Following are the transcripts of interviews with clinician experts who treat children with PANS/PANDAS/AE everyday. These are the clinicians working in the trenches and on the front lines with our sick kids. We interviewed a variety of different types of clinicians to allow for a broader perspective on the treatment options and approaches available to families today. No one clinician has all the answers, and each has had unique clinical experiences.

The following interviews do not constitute legal or medical advice, counseling, or other professional services and are not a substitute for professional diagnosis or treatment. You should always seek advice from a qualified health provider regarding a medical condition. If you have an emergency you should contact 911 or your doctor immediately. Do not disregard medical advice or delay seeking such advice based on the information found in this book.

WILLIAM LEE COWDEN, MD

Read excerpts from our interview with PANDAS and Lyme expert, Dr. William Lee Cowden. In this interview Dr. Cowden talks about how certain environmental assaults to the body (such as a chemical-toxin exposure, toxic mold exposure, or a physical head injury/concussion) can serve as a trigger and precursor to PANDAS/PANS symptoms. Typically the child's immune system is already under stress, is compromised, or his/her body has built up such a burden of stressors (toxic, emotional, microbial or other) that these events trigger a much worse cascade of illness than a child who is not carrying a substantial total body burden. Dr. Cowden's interview explains that while the microbes implicated in PANS (such as *Strep, Borrelia, Babesia,* etc.) are very important, whether or not a child succumbs to the syndrome of PANS/PANDAS and the severity of their symptoms may depend on what kind of toxic/inflammatory burden the child is already carrying.

What makes someone susceptible to PANDAS/PANS?; what do you think are some of the biggest issues that makes one vulnerable or susceptible to developing this condition?

There are a variety of things. For example, if somebody has had a previous concussive head injury, they're going to have an immune response to try to repair that concussive head injury. The immune system cells go into that area of the brain that's been injured, and those white blood cells have been scavenging toxins elsewhere in the body, and when the white cells end up in that area of the brain, trying to repair it, some of those white cells are going to die and deposit those toxins that are inside their bodies into that part of the brain. So then that part of the brain becomes more toxic than the other part of the brain, and if the toxins build up in that part of the brain because of that vicious cycle that gets going . . .with toxins causing microbes to grow. Microbes produce an inflammatory response, the immune system cytokine release. Then that causes blood vessel dilation, more white cells, cytokines, and so on.

The vicious cycle gets going and then before you know it, the patient's got a big load of microbes in their brain. You can get the same type of phenomena whenever a person has had a chemical exposure, and it doesn't have to be a man-made chemical. It can be a biotoxic chemical, like when a child living in a moldy environment breathes in mycotoxins, or sometimes mold and mycotoxins . . . and those mycotoxins can settle into an area of the brain that's active at that moment. So if a child is doing a visual task, and they're really studying hard on something visu-

ally, then those toxins are going to end up more in their occipital lobe of the brain than any other place in the brain.

If the child is focusing on trying to calculate a mathematical problem, it's going to show up in the frontal lobe of the brain where they do their mathematical calculations and so on. So different areas get affected in different levels. If the child's trying to understand speech or understand reading, it's going to settle into the temporal lobe, and so each child has a different presentation because of which areas of the brain that are most affected in them.

So the toxins and microbes will settle in the portion of the brain where the brain was active at the time the blood-brain barrier was breached?

Yes, so let's say that they go into the school room, the school room's got mold and fungus in it, and the first thing the teacher says is, "Get out your math book and do these problems on this page." So the child is busily working on the mathematical problems on that page, focusing a lot of blood flow and energy into the frontal lobe, and so that's where the mycotoxins are going to settle, in the frontal lobe.

So then you'll have sometimes the inability to do math after that because there's such a high level of toxins in the frontal lobe, and the microbes will settle into the frontal lobe because there's a high level of toxins there that create the environment that makes it easy for the microbes to thrive and survive and makes it hard for the white blood cells to survive to be able to eliminate the microbes.

What kinds of treatment modalities are most effective for PANS/PANDAS?

A lot of parents, unfortunately, look for the magic bullet. They want to just do one thing, and nothing but one thing, and get a miraculous cure. And sometimes that happens, but I think that it's very important for parents to look at the PANS and PAN-

DAS in more of a gestaltic fashion. Look at what is the whole picture. What was present when this started? What is still present now that could keep it going, and what can we get rid of that started it or kept it going? So is that the EMFs? Let's clean up the EMF environment. Is it the chemicals in the bedroom because you've got carpet and formaldehyde off-gassing from that, or fresh benzene, xylene, toluene in the paint in the wall? Or is it mold or fungus in the air conditioning system, or under the sink or wherever?

See, you want to try to look for all those things because I don't think you really make a huge impact on a chronic condition like PANS or PANDAS unless you address some of those causations. So the analogy that I make to patients is that everybody that's chronically ill is like a beast of burden that's walking down the path of life, and on either side of the path are workers bundling up bundles of straw, figuratively, and throwing them onto the beast of burden's back. Somewhere along the path, the beast of burden comes crashing to his or her knees, if they're out of the hospital, crashing to their belly if they're in the hospital, and a lot of the patients or the parents, will think, "Let's just take that last bundle off and get up." Well, no, it doesn't work that way. The beast of burden has to have almost the entire load taken off before they can even get up again.

What are some of the factors that make a child particularly susceptible to the development of PANDAS/PANS?

Many things: There's nutritional deficiencies. The kids nowadays don't go outside and play in the sunlight. They play on their computer games indoors. They get no sunlight exposure, no vitamin D production. For most of them, if they haven't been taking vitamin D as a supplement, their vitamin D levels are profoundly low. That has a huge impact on the immune system, on sugar metabolism, on calcium metabolism, magnesium uptake from the gut, and so many other things. Kids are not going out and grounding to the earth. They're sitting on synthetic ma-

terials in the house, with synthetic shoes on their feet, sleeping on synthetic beds at night, never grounding to the earth. What's that doing to us?

Editors Note: *It is important to remember that outdoor exposure might be less helpful if sunblock is applied as most sunblock prevents the skin experiencing the sun in a natural way. This can prevent vitamin D synthesis but can also interfere with other biological processes (such as the production of cholesterol sulfate and enzyme production) necessary for making energy and detoxifying.*

Of course, microbes such as *Strep*, Lyme, and Lyme co-infectors like *Babesia, Bartonella,* etc. are very important in the development of PANDAS/PANS symptoms, but do you think there can be too much emphasis on microbes and not enough emphasis on the host or terrain?

In most patients, most of the PANS symptoms are coming from the microbes, and toxins create an environment that allows the microbes to grow, so toxins are involved in that way. And it's not just the microbes, but it's also the biotoxins produced by the microbes. However, I think there is way too much emphasis on the microbe... if patients don't deal with the basics, working to get rid of the microbe is going to be a futile effort, I think, in most cases. Because even if they can get rid of the microbe for a time, it's only going to be for a time because the toxins that are there, the immune system that's suppressed, the nutritional deficiencies, etc., the strong EMF environment, all are going to create the environment to allow the microbe to rapidly recur. I don't think you can get rid of 100% of all microbes. You can get rid of a large percentage of microbes, but those that don't get killed off with whatever treatment regimen you're using are going to come back, as long as the circumstances are right for them to come back. And if you haven't done anything about the circumstances, they're going to come back.

And I would say that parents oftentimes want to get the biggest, meanest, ugliest bug killer that they can find to murder that bug, and oftentimes, they're doing the child a huge disservice because you could find an herbal product, for example, oftentimes, that will eliminate the bug just as well as those really powerful pharmaceutical antibiotics, without killing off every bug in the gut and destroying the immune system and creating leaky gut, creating allergy reactions in the brain and all the downstream impact.

There's a huge gut-brain connection, and if you make the gut worse, you're going to make the brain worse, and is that what they want? There are ways to get rid of the bugs with alcoholic tinctures of herbals without having hardly any adverse effect on the gut. Why wouldn't they do that instead of taking the pharmaceutical tablet that is a powerful bug killer, rolling down through the gut, killing every bug in sight before it finally gets absorbed?

Why do you believe herbal tinctures may be a better choice than pharmaceutical antibiotics?

Well, most antibiotics that are given by doctors in the United States are tablets. They're tablets of a strong pharmaceutical antibacterial antimicrobial, and those tablets don't break down in the stomach and get absorbed out of the stomach. They break down really slowly as they roll down through the small and large intestine. So somewhere down there, probably in the distal small intestine, they finally get completely broken down and absorbed, but they killed billions of bugs, friendly bugs in the gut as they get to that place where it's finally absorbed. When you take the alcoholic tinctures of herbs, it's rare when you see any of that making it into the second part of the small intestine. It's being absorbed in the stomach and duodenum, by energetic testing, at least, and almost none of it making it into the small intestine where it could kill friendly bacteria.

Capsules are better than tablets, for sure, but alcoholic tinctures are better than capsules because you're going to get an absorption higher up in the gut. You know, a lot of people use Iodoral, which is a tableted iodine product, and that kills lots and lots and lots of friendly bacteria in the gut as it rolls through there, waiting to be absorbed. So why don't we instead use Lugol's iodine solution and absorb it out of the stomach and not let it get into the small intestine and kill friendly bacteria there.

What effect do EMFs (electromagnetic fields from modern living) have on PANDAS/PANS?

Electromagnetic fields are known to disrupt the blood-brain barrier, but that'll cause a global brain effect. That'll cause the toxins that are in the bloodstream at that moment to go through the blood-brain barrier, or what used to be the blood-brain barrier into the brain, and create an environment that allows microbes to grow throughout the brain.

What role does emotional trauma or emotional stress play in PANDAS/PANS?

If a child is made to feel stupid by a teacher or by a parent about a certain thing, then that's what we call a conflict of perceived evaluation. That perceived evaluation will cause toxins to accumulate in the part of the brain that was involved in that particular event. So the parent says, or the school teacher says, "Couldn't you see that?" Figuratively, couldn't you see that? So that shows up in the occipital lobe. Or, "I can't believe you performed so poorly on that sporting event." That's going to show up in the parietal lobe. That's the motor cortex. Or you know, "I can't believe that you couldn't figure that out." That will show up in the frontal lobe.

Editor's Note: *Here Dr. Cowden is explaining how the type of emotional trauma or stress experienced at the time of a toxin/chemical or other exposure may actually direct where in the brain the microbes and toxins may accumulate. So if the child is*

*activating a portion of the brain that has to do with "sight" (liter-
ally or figuratively) then they may accumulate toxins in the portion of the brain that deals with sight (so the occipital lobe), or
if a child is activating a portion of the brain that has to do with
motor function, they may accumulate toxins/microbes in the parietal lobe (which is involved in sensory and motor function).*

How would you describe the perfect healing environment for a child with PANDAS/PANS?

*I would say the very most important is the emotional envi-
ronment. If the parents are toxic, then they're going to have a
toxic child. So it's really important for the parents to keep in
mind that they could be doing ongoing damage to the child, just
by the way that they react to the child. They need to learn how
to become unconditionally loving without having any criticism,
all that kind of stuff, if they can, because again, that impacts the
brain and how the toxins are taken up into the brain.*

*I think the second greatest impact is the electromagnetic en-
vironment, so getting rid of the WiFi, the cordless phone, the cell
phone, putting it on airplane mode, turning off the breaker that
goes to the bedroom at night, you know, getting rid of the electric
SmartMeter if it's too close to the bedroom, et cetera. All those
EMF things, to the best of your ability. We live in an imperfect
world, so we can't get rid of all of it unless you move out into the
countryside, you can. But most people don't have the luxury of
living in the countryside and working in the city.*

Can you talk a bit about how you use photonic enhanced uptake with infrared light along with herbals?

*We use infrared-light-emitting diodes. When you shine an in-
frared light into the tissue, it stimulates the production of nitric
oxide. Nitric oxide relaxes the smooth circumferential muscles
in the arterials, which then dilates the blood vessels and allows
more blood supply into that area, so if you've got herbs in the
blood stream at that moment, then more herb is going to come
to that place than any other place in the body.*

What would you say is the most common mistake that parents make when they are trying to help their child heal from PANDAS or PANS?

Well, I think it is when you focus on one bug and not looking at the whole picture well enough. If they'll look at the whole picture and start addressing enough of the causations, then they don't have to focus nearly as hard on the one bug.

What advice would you give to a parent who has a child with a new PANDAS/PANS diagnosis who is expressing psychiatric symptoms?

If it's a psychiatric manifestation, my advice would be: Do not put them on a psychiatric drug. That's the worst thing that they could do, in my opinion. And it's not that I have a lot of animosity toward psychiatric drugs, but I just don't think that they work very well, and if they do work, it's going to take two weeks for them to work. But in natural medicine, we have ways to get an improvement in a child's psychiatric condition in hours to days, rather than weeks to months. Why don't we do those things first?

Most of the herbals that I use have proven anti-inflammatory effects. We know that a lot of what goes on with the neuropsychiatric conditions is an inflammatory process in the brain. Well, why don't we use something that's going to have maybe a little antimicrobial effect, quite a bit of anti-inflammatory effect, and not damage the friendly bacteria in the gut, not cause leaky gut, not cause food allergy reactions, not cause all the other complications that you get with the pharmaceutical drugs or the adverse effects that you get on screwing up the neurotransmitters and the neurotransmitter receptors that you get with psychiatric drugs? Why don't we use some of those simpler, less-risky, in most cases less-expensive modalities first?

Any final words of wisdom, Dr. Cowden?

Well, I think another really important thing is for the message to get out that when an allopathic doctor says there is nothing else that can be done, that's an incorrect statement. What their statement should be is, "I know of nothing else that can be done. Go search on your own, or go find an integrative practitioner that can help you find other answers. Okay?" But it just irks me completely, to no end, when an allopathic doctor says there is no more hope, because the most important factor in getting well is hope.

ELENA FRID, MD

Dr. Elena Frid is a Board Certified Neurologist and Clinical Neurophysiologist diagnostician, advisor, and a treatment strategist specializing in Infections Induced Autoimmune Disorders. In addition to practicing general neurology, Dr. Frid also focuses on Autoimmune, Neurodegenerative, and Neuropsychiatric disorders which includes Lyme and associated co-infections, autoimmune encephalitis, CFS, PANDAS/PANS, dementias and other. In 2011, Dr. Frid opened her solo practice in New York City conveniently located in the heart of Manhattan where she sees both children and adult patients. Using cutting-edge diagnostic tools and clinical expertise, she differentiates between idiopathic vs. organic causes of various neurological disorders. Her knowledge has been sought by patients from all over the United States, Canada, and Europe. Dr. Frid is a member of the American Academy of Neurology (AAN). She is a voting member of the International Lyme and Associated Diseases Society (ILADS), Vice President of Robert Wood Johnson Medical School Alumni Association, and a member of the Independent Physicians of New York (IDNY). You can follow Dr. Frid on Facebook and Instagram @drelenafrid where she raises awareness for the above conditions. Sign up to her website newsletter: www.ElenaFridMD.com for updates on latest medical information and events. You can also follow her on her YouTube channel: Lyme Talk with Dr. Frid.

What laboratory tests or non-laboratory assessments, if any, do you recommend for patients diagnosed with PANDAS/PANS/AE?

I look at PANDAS/PANS as falling under the Autoimmune Encephalitis umbrella, which is when you have an inflammation and autoimmune process that creates antineuronal antibodies changing the brain matrix and in turn creating neuropsychiatric symptoms in some instances. In my practice I use an Autoimmune Encephalitis panel from the Mayo Clinic which includes looking for NMDA receptor antibodies, K+ channel receptor antibodies, GAD65-receptor antibodies assessed in blood and cerebrospinal fluid, as well as the use of the Cunningham Panel in serum. I also recommend patients obtain brain imaging such as MRI of the head, Brain SPECT scan, an EEG and neurocognitive assessment done with a neuropsychiatrist in order to assess the level of impairment that the patient is presenting with.

What kinds of treatment modalities are most effective for treating PANDAS/PANS/AE?

The treatment modalities depend on the underlying cause of the autoimmune encephalitis. If one has identified an infectious etiology for the presentation that is thought to be triggering the autoimmune phenomenon, in this case one should be treating the underlying infection. A patient is then monitored closely and if he/she is not showing significant progress, it would be appropriate to introduce immune-modulating therapy such as IVIG to help modulate the immune system and quiet down the immune response that is causing an insult to the central nervous system.

What diet and lifestyle modifications are most important for children experiencing symptoms of PANDAS/PANS/AE?

Some patients report improvement of symptoms on an anti-inflammatory diet. I must say that often when symptoms are very pronounced, diet modifications are minimally effective and focusing only on dietary changes and restrictions becomes frustrating both to the patient and the family.

If you could describe the perfect healing environment for a child with PANDAS/PANS/AE, what would it look like?

I often explain to families as well as educators that children with Autoimmune Encephalitis should be treated like a Traumatic Brain Injury patient. One must be aware that these children have a continuous insult to their brain. The recommendations to each patient are individual based on their level of functioning. However, overall if a child is only able to tolerate part-time school or minimal physical activity, I recommend they do a certain amount of work daily, enough so that they are not recovering from a specific activity for multiple hours or days. If they are not functional after an activity for prolonged period of time, they should cut back on exposure enough so that it does not wipe them out fully.

What is the most common mistake parents of children with PANDAS/PANS/AE make along their healing journey?

A common mistake is that the symptoms are not addressed early enough in the disease process because they can be very subtle and build up over time. No one knows your child better than you do! If he/she is exhibiting a change in their behavior such as unexplained anxiety, becoming a picky eater, regression of behavior, bedwetting, vocal or motor tics, fatigue, gastrointestinal problems, pain and more, see a specialist as it is easier to treat and cure autoimmune encephalitis early on in the disease process. Please note that your child does not have to present with all these symptoms, and they may have additional symptoms that are not mentioned above.

What is the best piece of advice you would give a parent whose neurotypical child is "suddenly crazy"... a child that develops neuropsychiatric symptoms out of the blue?

Parents need to know that infections, inflammatory processes as well as autoimmune disorders, and other medical problems can trigger neuropsychiatric symptoms. When addressing just the psychiatric part of the presentation with psychotropic medications, one maybe be missing the underlying cause of the disease process and in turn prolong the suffering of the patient and the family, and it makes it more difficult to treat and cure the condition. Please see a physician who specializes in Autoimmune Encephalitis if you suspect that as a diagnosis as this is a complex medical problem that needs to be addressed promptly and appropriately for best outcomes.

TOM MOORCROFT, DO

Dr. Tom Moorcroft is a global leader in solving complex medical mysteries. He completed his undergraduate studies at the University of Vermont before attending the University of New England College of Osteopathic Medicine (UNECOM). While at UNECOM, Tom was selected to complete a one-year fellowship in Osteopathic Manipulative Medicine. Tom completed his residency training in Family Medicine at Middlesex Hospital in Middletown, CT. Dr. Tom is board certified in Family Medicine and Osteopathic Manipulative Treatment. He is a co-founder of Origins of Health, an Osteopathic wellness center, focused on solving the riddles of chronic illness to enable their patients to regain their health and regain their lives. Dr. Moorcroft specializes in the diagnosis and treatment of chronic tick-borne illness, mold illness and Infections-Induced Autoimmune Encephalitis in children and adults. Learn more about Dr. Moorcroft at www.OriginsOfHealth.com

What laboratory tests or non-laboratory assessments, if any, do you recommend for patients diagnosed with PANDAS/PANS/AE?

I start with a comprehensive history and physical exam to help determine the most appropriate testing strategy. I recommend testing for potential underlying causes of the patient's symptoms. This should include checking for possible infectious triggers, such as tick-borne infections, Bartonella, Streptococcus, Mycoplasma and Chlamydia pneumoniae, Candida, and viruses. Evaluation of baseline immune system function should be done, checking for immunoglobulins, particularly IgA, IgG and IgM levels, and mannose-binding lectin. An autoimmune neurology panel, offered at most conventional labs, can rule in or out other possible causes of Autoimmune Encephalitis. A Cunningham panel should be considered to evaluate for presence of antineuronal antibodies.

What kinds of treatment modalities are most effective for treating PANDAS/PANS/AE?

Identifying the underlying cause or trigger of the symptoms is paramount. Once the underlying cause or causes are identified, I find an integrative approach to treatment is most effective. This may include pharmaceutical or natural antibiotics, antifungals, and/or anti-parasitics (medications and herbals). In my practice, I find most patients need a combination of both approaches at some point during their treatment. I rarely see just herbs or just medications getting the job done. In addition to treatment of the underlying infection, I find support of detoxification and modulation of the immune system are required. The starting point for this is gut support - improving the diet, removing foods that may be adding to inflammation (including simple sugars, processed foods and potentially gluten and dairy), supporting daily bowel movements, etc. Depending upon one's age, the gastrointestinal tract houses 50-70% of your immune cells. Modulation of the immune response starts with

*healing the gut. Interestingly, a significant amount of gut dys-
function is caused by infections in the gut wall, so the combination of anti-infective treatments and dietary changes can be a
potent one-two punch.*

*In some situations, the autoimmune reaction triggered by the
infections or other underlying cause is so intense that IVIG and/
or a steroid taper are required. It is also critical to evaluate for
other potential triggers and contributing factors. Any internal
or external stressor on the body can cause inflammation leading to worsening of symptoms. Your body has an amazing self-
healing mechanism, but at times it gets overwhelmed. It is our
job to determine what are the major issues impeding the work
of the self-healing mechanism and help to remove them. Many
times I find that the issue that is preventing healing is not the
initial trigger of the Autoimmune Encephalitis. Many times,
providers are so focused on treating infections or modulating
an over-reactive immune system that they miss other major im-
pediments to healing, such as emotional traumas, social stressors, structural changes, or poor diet. The most important piece
of this puzzle is determining the body's healing priorities, to the
best of our abilities, and supporting the work of the self-healing
mechanism, specifically in these areas. Once we know what the
diagnosis is, choosing the appropriate treatment modality becomes much easier.*

Can you talk a bit about the physical structure of the body and how structural integrity is an important, but often overlooked, part of healing and wellness? (especially with regard to PANDAS/PANS/AE)

*The underlying physiologic functions of the human body pre-
exist its physical form. These functions dictate the development
and appearance of the human form. This phenomena is often
described as form follows function. In other words, we look the
way we do in order for our bodies to function as they should.
During development, organs and tissues frequently start devel-*

opment in one area of the body then migrate to another bringing along with them nerves, blood vessels, and connective tissues. What this means for us is that muscles in our backs have a direct connection to internal organs, such as the heart, liver, kidneys and gastrointestinal tract. Changes in internal organs can lead to changes in the muscles, and changes in the muscles can lead to changes in the function of the internal organs. This dynamic inter-relationship gives the osteopathic physician unique insights into the cause of illness as well as the ability to apply osteopathic manipulative treatments to help alleviate a significant amount of our patient's suffering.

Dr. A.T. Still, MD, DO, founder of Osteopathic Medicine, became famous by treating cholera, a type of infectious diarrhea, with osteopathic manipulation, a gentle, hands-on form of diagnosis and treatment. Additionally, in our current era of less-than-optimal diets, many of my patients have underdeveloped airways, crooked teeth, open bites and mouth breathing. All of these can lead to decreased oxygen getting to their developing brains. I have many children with night sweats, tic disorders and behavioral abnormalities who realize dramatic improvements, if not complete resolution of symptoms, when their orofacial structural abnormalities are addressed. Instead of antibiotics and IVIG, these children work with a functional dentist, a myofunctional therapist (essentially a physical therapist for the mouth and tongue) and an osteopathic physician who specializes in osteopathic manipulative treatment. These patients may also need other interventions, such as antimicrobial treatments and dietary modifications, but addressing their underlying structural issues improves oxygenation and eases physical strains on their developing brains, which in turn leads to less inflammation, less symptoms and improved overall health and development.

If you could describe the perfect healing environment for a child with PANDAS/PANS/AE, what would it look like?

I think a perfect healing environment is difficult to describe because every child must be treated as the unique individual they are, and what is perfect for one child may not be perfect for another. I believe the most important factors are love and compassion. Patients and their parents have a need to receive as well as give love, be treated with compassion and feel appreciated. A loving, supportive environment is crucial. I recommend a well-balanced lifestyle and environment. This should include family time, including meals with a whole-food, plant-based diet balanced with meats, fats and appropriate grains.

An environment free of external toxins, such as molds and negative electromagnetic fields (EMFs), is also important. In this day and age where everything is becoming more and more high-tech and wireless, we are all exposed to the negative effects of EMFs. The negative effects of EMFs are many, and the list continues to grow. Some of the symptoms reported from high EMF exposure include: increased anxiety, sensation of your skin crawling, brain fog, poor sleep, and generalized inflammation.

One simple trick to improve sleep and decrease body-wide inflammation is to turn off your WiFi at night. Simply put your WiFi router on a timer, set it and forget it. Within a week or two you'll be amazed how much better everyone in the house is sleeping, and the change it will likely have on your child's behavior.

An outdoor environment is also critical for the growth and development of children as well as their recovery. Everyone needs some fresh air - go outside and play, open the windows and air the house out for a few minutes a day, even in the winter. Movement is essential for healing. The primary mechanism for clearing toxins in the arms and legs is muscle contraction. In the chest and abdomen, it is pressure-gradient changes caused by deep breathing. Running around and playing are key com-

ponents of overall body detoxification and immune system support. Sleep is a critical component to health. The mechanisms of brain detoxification function primarily during deep sleep. Creating a sleep sanctuary that minimizes screens, lights, or EMFs, especially in the evening, is an important component to your child's healing.

As I mentioned, balance is key. The sicker someone is, the more strict they may need to be in order to heal, but don't forget to allow your kid to be a kid. Trying to do everything perfectly can create a lot of unnecessary stress for you and your child. No need to create even more inflammation. Treat your child and yourself with compassion by keeping the principle of balance in mind.

What is the most common mistake parents of children with PANDAS/PANS/AE make along their healing journey?

There are so many challenges that face parents of a child with PANDAS/PANS/AE. The parents I work with are usually willing to do anything possible to help their child. In their search for health, parents frequently seek advice from anywhere they can find it. This often leads to seeing three, four, five, even 10 or more providers looking for answers. They end up mixing bits and pieces of different treatment protocols, and then they get mixed results. This leads to second guessing their providers and themselves. In turn, they start seeking more advice and adding more things into the treatment protocol. I can't tell you how many times, at the end of an appointment, a parent says, "oh, I almost forgot to tell you I added xyz supplement because I read it might help." I also see children having tremendous flares of their symptoms that I am having a hard time managing only to find out weeks later that the child was started on three or four new treatments that I was not told about. I recommend parents find a provider they are comfortable with and work with them. Follow their protocol. Realize that doing too many different things or taking bits and pieces from different protocols typi-

cally doesn't work. Have an open and honest relationship with your provider. If you feel you want to try something different, ask that person. I'm often happy to have a patient try something I'm not totally familiar with as long as I know the person supervising that aspect of treatment is well-trained in its use and I know when the change is being made. I commonly work with a team of providers, but there does need to be one provider who is at the helm making sure all the treatments are working together rather than being counter-productive.

Another mistake I see relates to time: not waiting long enough to allow the treatments to work or staying on the same treatments forever even though they are not working. It is so difficult to have patience when you child is suffering. Symptoms will commonly wax and wane in frequency and intensity as a part of the natural history of PANDAS/PANS/AE. Your child will have good days and bad days. A bad day does not necessarily mean the treatment protocol needs to be changed, just as one good day amongst many bad days does not mean the protocol is working well. Unfortunately, we cannot always fix a bad day, and your child may suffer more than any of us would like. This is often the case due a Herxheimer-type or die-off reaction. This is a sign the treatment protocol is working, but for a period of time symptoms will be worse before getting better. Looking at the trend of symptoms over time in conjunction with your main provider is the best way to determine when changes need to be made.

What is the best piece of advice you would give a parent whose neurotypical child is "suddenly crazy"... a child that develops neuropsychiatric symptoms out of the blue?

Neuro-psychiatric symptoms out of the blue are not normal. This may seem obvious, but I commonly see previously healthy children told they have acute-onset OCD at age nine with no previous personal or family history of mental health issues. Do the best you can to have your child evaluated immediately. Common triggers for these acute onset events include streptococ-

cal and tick-borne infections. Look for other symptoms, such as throat pain, joint pains, rashes, that you can point out to your child's doctor. I've been pleasantly surprised how many more providers are aware of the possibility of PANDAS/PANS/AE over the past several years. When you present your concerns, it may be helpful to provide them information on PANDAS/PANS/AE. Doctors tend to be more open to information from sources they are familiar with. Medical literature or publications from organizations with respected doctors on their advisory boards are good bets. Print-outs from chat groups or someone's personal blog generally do not hold as much weight with doctors. There are few faster ways to turn off a doctor than to tell them how to do their job based upon what you read on the internet. Establish a relationship with a good pediatrician now. If your child's doctor knows them and your family before anything happens, they will have a better likelihood of seeing changes in your child and believing you because you have a long-standing relationship. In an acute-onset event, it is important to act quickly. If you notice something is wrong, call your doctor immediately. In terms of PANDAS/PANS/AE, it may be difficult to get someone to listen. Contact one of the reputable PANDAS/PANS/AE organizations for a physician referral.

Why do you think we are seeing so many cases of sudden onset PANDAS/PANS/AE in children right now?

The amount and intensity of stressors we are all exposed today likely plays a big role. Technology has led to us being exposed to more EMFs and negative content than ever before. These stressors lead to tremendous inflammation in our bodies. Our food supply is becoming less and less nutritious due to poor farming practices and introduction of genetically modified foods. The widespread use of pesticides and other chemicals also exert tremendous pressures on our bodies and our food supply. In general, children are more sedentary than when I was a kid. Less activity and poor food choices have led to obesity and hormone imbalances. Lack of exercise diminishes the efficacy of the body's primary detoxification pathways. Children and adults are complaining of sleep disturbances more than ever before. As about 90% of the brain's detoxification occurs during slow-wave sleep, anything that interferes with our normal sleep schedule can potentially increase the baseline inflammation in our brains. This includes EMFs, screen time and lights later in the evening, and racing minds from an overly stressful lifestyle. More children and adults are likely developing Autoimmune Encephalitis because of the dramatic increase in the toxic loads we are exposed to on a daily basis. Our baseline levels of stress and inflammation are higher in turn leading to a decreased level of immune system health.

Prevention is key. While you are not likely going to be able to prevent your child from being exposed to Streptococcus, you can help them achieve a higher level of baseline balance and health in their lives. Start by making sleep, healthy eating and spending quality time together priorities. Decrease exposure to artificial lights and EMFs, particularly at night. Limit screen time. Make it a point to get outside and move together. Take a moment each day to realize how awesome it is to be alive and how incredible your body's self-healing mechanism is. Model these behaviors for your child and see their and your health improve.

ROSEANN CAPANNA-HODGE, EdD, LPC, BCN

Dr. Roseann Capanna-Hodge is a Connecticut Certified School Psychologist, a Licensed Professional Counselor (LPC) and a Board Certified Neurofeedback Provider (BCN), with more than 20 years working with children, teens, adults and parents. She answered her calling to be a psychologist and currently has private practice offices in Ridgefield and Newtown, CT, where the focus is on neurofeedback, biofeedback, counseling and assessment for a variety of issues and conditions. After seeing individuals and families suffer through unsuccessful attempts at traditional therapies, Dr. Roseann became passionate about using highly effective research-based, non-medication and brain-based therapies to alleviate stress and suffering, bringing children and adults to a point of wellness. She uses neuroscience bridged with clinical therapies to address a variety of issues. Dr. Roseann specializes in anxiety and anxiety-related disorders, ADHD, autism, executive functioning, dyslexia and other reading disabilities, learning disabilities, Lyme and tick-borne disease, PANS/PANDAS, concussion/postconcussion syndrome and parent coaching.

What laboratory tests or non-laboratory assessments, if any, do you recommend for patients diagnosed with PANDAS/PANS/AE?

In conjunction with a detailed clinical intake, a QEEG (Quantitative Electroencephalography) brain map assesses the impact of infectious disease on brain-wave functioning. A QEEG also determines an individual's neurocognitive and neuropsychological functioning. This simple process involves putting on a cap, taking a measurement of one's brainwaves, and comparing that data to a database. From there, you can see patterns associated with certain conditions and issues and then understand where dysregulation is in the brain. It provides a wealth of information about their neurocognitive functioning. A QEEG helps us understand the real issues leading to better treatment recommendations and can give a wealth of information to better support a child with PANS/PANDAS.

Additionally, behavioral ratings analyze issues from a more behavioral perspective. Again, this identifies core issues. For example, one person may express focus issues as difficulty completing tasks and another person may see focus issues as being easily distracted. Without identifying the true behavior, treatment and progress cannot be measured effectively. Traditional mental health procedures lack scientific assessments when diagnosing issues, as they just refer to the Diagnostic and Statistical Manual (DSM) to compare symptoms. To date, the available genetic testing that examines common mutations associated with mental health issues is not the norm. Using QEEG and behavioral ratings should be the standard in mental health, not only for diagnostic reasonings but also for measuring treatment outcomes.

What kinds of treatment modalities are most effective for treating PANDAS/PANS/AE?

In terms of mental health treatments for PANS, a variety of supportive holistic, clinical treatments exists. Psychotherapy and psychoeducation are essential. Parents need psychoeducation about ways the disease impacts the neurological and behavioral factors. Moreover, they need direct coaching on managing the behaviors associated with PANS including but not limited to OCD, tics, rage, emotional lability, and anxiety. Parents need guidance and support to help them handle the intensity of the behaviors.

Therapies to calm the central nervous system help the body and brain heal. Additionally, Cognitive Behavior Therapy (CBT) and Exposure and Response Prevention therapy (ERP) teach the child to better respond to behaviors associated with PANS. Holistic and research-based therapies, such as neurofeedback, biofeedback, PEMF, hypnosis, EFT/tapping, EMDR, and reiki are effective because they work at the subconscious level. During high levels of flare activation, kids with PANDAS/PANS aren't present enough to do talk therapy, so subconscious therapies can reduce symptoms without requiring the child to exert effort. Living through the turmoil of a flare requires relief and therapies that calm the central nervous system without adding stress. Once the central nervous system is calm and symptoms are reduced enough for a child to engage in talk therapy, then CBT or ERP can further support the reduction of symptoms, such as: obsessions and compulsions, anxiety, depression, anger, executive functioning and attention, managing emotions and so on.

What diet and lifestyle modifications are most important for children experiencing symptoms of PANDAS/PANS/AE?

An anti-inflammatory diet, as well as lifestyle changes incorporating sleep and reducing stress are the cornerstones of healing a child with PANDAS/PANS. While these seem overwhelming to parents, they need to happen. In addition to diet and lifestyle changes, parents should identify genetic issues and nutrient deficiencies to further their child's healing.

If you could describe the perfect healing environment for a child with PANDAS/PANS/AE, what would it look like?

Patience and persistence act as the foundation to heal a PANDAS/PANS child. Combining diet and lifestyle modifications with traditional and holistic treatments aids long-term, chronic cases. Ideally, parents should homeschool children while they are healing to reduce infectious disease exposure and generally reduce stress. Moreover, homeschooling offers the flexibility needed for provider appointments as well as greater consistency when using supplements and homeopathy.

What is the most common mistake parents of children with PANDAS/PANS/AE make along their healing journey?

Parents of children with PANDAS/PANS find the foundational pieces (diet, lifestyle, sleep, genetic issues, and nutrient deficiencies) most challenging. These often involve changes for the whole family. Also, the desire for a healthy child makes the often long and uncharted treatment process frustrating. PANS/PANDAS drains parent energy and leaves many parents without the necessary energy or support. Working on the foundational pieces while incorporating medical or other treatments can seem overwhelming to parents when also helping children struggling to heal but are necessary elements. There isn't a stand-alone treatment that is curative at this time, which is frustrating, but a combined approach can bring healing.

What is the best piece of advice you would give a parent whose neurotypical child is "suddenly crazy" and develops neuropsychiatric symptoms out of the blue?

The best piece of advice is to get to a PANS/PANDAS-literate physician and/or provider as quickly as you can. A sudden onset of psychiatric symptoms is completely abnormal, meaning a root cause always exists. As soon as the child presents with neuropsychiatric symptoms, parents should obtain antimicrobial and antiviral support to mitigate acute symptoms and hopefully prevent chronic cases. Since PANS/PANDAS is an infectious disease, psychiatric medication will only delay proper treatment and not help. Working with PANS/PANDAS-literate mental health professionals and other providers who can help you through the healing process is essential. No one ever says, "I regret getting help right away", so don't delay when there is a sudden onset of psychiatric symptoms or a waxing or waning of symptoms.

VICTORIA KOBLINER, MS, RDN

Ms. Kobliner is a Registered Dietitian with years of expertise in applying a functional approach to nutrition. She develops individualized plans for clients that are designed to promote wellness, prevent disease and rebalance underlying nutritional impairments. A key element of this approach is the optimization of digestive function. Research shows that impairments in this critical nutritional pathway can have a far-reaching impact on our brain, immune, detoxification, and other seemingly unrelated systems. Ms. Kobliner has extensive experience in using dietary modification, appropriate supplementation and functional lab testing to achieve optimal wellness.

What are the most common symptoms of PANDAS/PANS/Autoimmune Encephalitis that you see in your practice?

Many of the symptoms we see are those that are consistent with the stressful impact that chronic inflammation can cause, but when they occur seemingly overnight, that is the hallmark of PANDAS/PANS. Often we see anxiety, anorexia, OCD, deterioration in school performance, aggression, sleep disturbance, changes in handwriting and/or anorexia. When all or some of these symptoms present suddenly in a child who was previously unaffected, that is an important clue.

What laboratory tests or non-laboratory assessments, if any, do you recommend for patients diagnosed with PANDAS/PANS/AE?

As with all the people we see, a thorough medical history is the essential first step. Determining if onset was acute or chronic is important in this interview. Appropriate tests to rule out other causes such as Tourette, Sydenham Chorea, etc., are indicated, as well. Strep titers such as ASO, DNase B, testing for Lyme and coinfections, immunoglobulin levels and a Cunningham panel can all help with diagnosis.

What kinds of treatment modalities are most effective for treating PANDAS/PANS/Autoimmune Encephalitis?

According to the 2017 Overview of Treatment of Pediatric Acute-Onset Neuropsychiatric Syndrome (Swedo, et al.), treating PANS requires a three-step approach which must always include three components.

1. *Treating the symptoms with modalities such as psychoactive medication, behavioral therapy and other supports.*

2. *Removing the source of the infection with antimicrobial therapy.*

3. *Immunomodulating and anti-inflammatory interventions to support a normal immune system.*

As a Registered Dietitian, I utilize antimicrobial and anti-inflammatory interventions such as diet and herbs/supplements. The specific diet and supplements recommended will always be specific to the individual.

What is the most common mistake parents of children with PANDAS/PANS/AE make along their healing journey?

I hesitate to say that parents are making mistakes on this journey- most of the time they are doing incredible things in the face of limited information, and an often unsupportive medical community, while watching a child suffer. However, expecting a quick response and therefore not sticking with treatment recommendations long enough is one challenge I see often.

What is the best piece of advice you would give a parent whose neurotypical child is "suddenly crazy"... a child that develops neuropsychiatric symptoms out of the blue?

Have them evaluated for PANS/PANDAS/AE with a knowledgeable specialist! Find support in PANS/PANDAS support groups, share your experience far and wide (you find information in the unlikeliest places), and never lose hope.

If you could describe the perfect healing environment for a child with PANDAS/PANS/Autoimmune Encephalitis what would it look like? (including nutritional, environmental, psychosocial, emotional and other forms of support)

An individualized approach is a must. It should incorporate appropriate medication to address underlying cause (bacterial, viral, etc.) as well as provide relief of acute emotional symptoms. An anti-inflammatory diet (individualized, especially if anorexia must be addressed), anti-inflammatory herbs/supplements, CBT therapy, support for family in home, educational and emotional support system for child at school. A home free of toxins from food as well as personal care and cleaning products will reduce the child's body burden. Avoid processed foods and sugars, which increase inflammation and deplete supportive nutrients. In other words, a lifestyle approach that nurtures the healing powers of the body while reducing the toxic burden we place on it works well.

LAUREN STONE, PhD, MS, HHP, BCIH

Lauren Stone is a nutritionist and holistic healthcare practitioner using BioEnergetic Medicine. Lauren came to BioEnergetic Medicine in the search to heal her own children, and chose to make it her career after experiencing its success first hand. In addition to a BA from Yale University and a PhD from Cornell University, Lauren has a Masters in Human Nutrition from the University of Bridgeport. She also holds an advanced certificate in BioSET, Quantum Reflex Analysis, and is a Board-Certified Holistic Health Practitioner, a Board-Certified Integrative Health Practitioner, a board member of Epidemic Answers, and a distinguished member of the American Association of Integrative Medicine.

Why do PANDAS/PANS/AE symptoms typically emerge in a child? What are the underlying physiological imbalances commonly seen in children presenting with symptoms of PANDAS/PANS/AE?

PANDAS/PANS/AE are all neurological manifestations of unchecked inflammation due to immune dysregulation. The infective process that is at the core of these syndromes is really just the proverbial "straw that broke the camel's back." In other words, children don't just suddenly wake up one day sick, although clinically this is how many affected kids present. Rather, PANDAS, PANS and AE are "total load syndromes." Like asthma and eczema and even autism, the immune system becomes so overwhelmed fending off everyday toxins in the form of the foods we eat and the air we breathe, that there is little energy

*left to effectively fight off microbial assaults when they occur.
Children affected by PANDAS/PANS/AE often present early
on with immune dysregulation in the form of allergies, asthma,
ADD/ADHD, eczema, gut dysfunction, and autism spectrum
disorders.*

Why are we seeing so many cases of sudden-onset PANDAS/PANS/AE in children right now?

*We live in a toxic world – the food we eat is laced with pes-
ticides, chemicals and artificial hormones. The air we breathe
and the water we drink are likewise contaminated. Our children
are the canaries in the coal mine, and the myriad of disorders
affecting them is the physiological expression of these ongoing,
toxic exposures.*

What are your thoughts on the role of the "microbe" versus the "terrain" in children with PANDAS/PANS/AE? Why is so much emphasis placed on killing/eradicating infectious agents (Lyme and coinfectors, *Strep, Mycoplasma,* etc.) in cases of PANDAS/PANS/AE?

*It is impossible to effectively fight the microbe without first
addressing the terrain. The ecology of the human body, when
functioning properly, is innately intelligent and always seeks
homeostasis, or balance. Many modern Western medical interventions, although valuable in their own right, have unwittingly
disrupted this balance, predisposing our children to a variety of
chronic illnesses.*

What diet and lifestyle modifications are most important for children experiencing symptoms of PANDAS/PANS/AE?

*Reducing inflammation is the first order of business when
fighting any chronic illness. This means reducing inflammatory
exposures whenever possible. Cleaning up the diet is typically a
great place to start. This includes eliminating foods that cause*

reactivity (wheat, dairy, soy and corn are generally the biggest culprits), eating organically whenever possible, and eating fresh, vibrant foods (not packaged foods from the grocery store). Cleaning up the home environment is also crucial – reducing or eliminating such toxic exposures as mold and EMF's is often an overlooked, but elemental, part of the healing process.

What is the role of the family in the treatment of a child with PANDAS/PANS/AE? Would you recommend that the entire family be treated, and if so, how?

Microbes are often passed between family members, even pets. Everyone should be checked and treated appropriately. Lifestyle changes should likewise be adopted by all.

TOBY WATKINSON, DC

Dr. Toby Watkinson has been in practice for 33 years, and at Scripps Medical Offices for the past 11 years. Dr. Watkinson grew up in Newport, Rhode Island, where his father was an innovative health practitioner who developed a practice that incorporated natural and holistic methods of healing. Dr. Watkinson graduated from Trinity University with a degree in Experimental and Physiological Psychology. For eight years, Dr. Watkinson worked as a research psychologist on contract for the Aerospace Medicine Research Laboratory, the Flight Dynamics Laboratory, and the Human Performance Laboratory at McDonnell Douglas Astronautics. As a continuation of his education, Dr. Watkinson completed his Doctorate in Chiropractic, earned a Board Certification in Clinical Thermography, a Certification in Acupuncture, and a Board Certification in Clinical Nutrition from the International and American Board of Clinical Nutrition. Dr. Watkinson is the past president and past vice-president of the International and American Association of Clinical Nutritionists. He served on the advisory board of the Price Pottenger Nutritional Foundation, and presently serves on the Advisory Board of the International Foundation of Health and Nutrition.

**Editor's Note: *In the following interview, some of Dr. Watkinson's responses are highly technical and/or complex in their medical explanation. In such cases, we have provided some notes to simplify the concept for the reader's benefit.*

Why do you think we're seeing so many cases of sudden onset PANS in children right now?

*I'm going to start with some very basic information, and that is that the brain rests at 7 to 8 Hz (Hertz). [**Editor's Note:** Like sound frequencies, brainwaves are measured in Hz, or cycles per second, so 7 Hz is equivalent to 7 cycles per second. An awake brain usually cycles at 8 to 25Hz or between 8 and 25 cycles per second.] These kids are being exposed to either 2.4 or 5 GHz— which translates to 2.4 to 5 billion cycles per second—from WiFi nearly 24/7.[54] So you figure if you live in an apartment complex or a condo complex or even in a neighborhood where the homes are together, you're going to have anywhere from two to five to eight WiFi routers in your face all the time, and that puts these children at risk, at great risk.*

Some of the studies that have been done at Yale have shown that if they take pregnant mice and they put cellphones on top of the cages of these pregnant mice that when these mice are born, they are hyperactive, and they can't memorize anything. They can't memorize running down a pathway and figuring which way to turn over and over again.[55]

*Well, why that happens is because cell phones/WiFi keeps you in a sympathetic state and a repressed parasympathetic state. [**Editor's Note:** The sympathetic nervous system is what dominates intense physical activity. It is the state we are in when we are scared or in "fight or flight" mode. The parasympathetic nervous system is dominant when we are in "relaxed" mode. This is also when our body does most of its repair and healing. If you are always in a sympathetic state, and never in a parasympa-*

---

54 https://www.ncbi.nlm.nih.gov/pubmed/25775055
55 https://www.nature.com/articles/srep00312

thetic state, your body cannot heal. Dr. Watkinson is explaining how exposure to WiFi/cell phones upregulates or triggers the sympathetic nervous system and downregulates or represses the parasympathetic nervous system.[56]] In other words, you have no brakes and you have all gas pedal, and what that equates to is a failure of digestion and a turning off of your immune system. What it does with most of these folks is put them into nearly a constant hyper-vigilant state where they never really relax and never truly repair or heal.

Can you talk about pathogens and how the immune system of these kids cannot effectively eradicate them?

There are some microbial or toxic exposures that are especially dangerous, and one is mycotoxin. Mycotoxin is not well known by a lot of people. When most people think of mycotoxin, they think "oh, that's some sort of mold thing." Well, it is some sort of mold thing, but mycotoxin can actually live on after the mold is no longer there. We can inhale it. It goes through our lungs, but it doesn't stay there, it stays in the gut where, because of the connection between the lymphatic tissue in the gut and the brain, you can end up with mycotoxin in your brain, which can look like symptoms of Huntington's, or it can look like myasthenia gravis, it looks like all these other (neurological or behavioral) conditions, but it's really mycotoxin.

*Now, what happens with mycotoxin is it puts us into kind of a TH17 state (a state where TH17 cells proliferate, associated with autoimmune disease) in which the body's immune response cannot deal with it the way that it should to get rid of it. [**Editor's Note:** TH17 cell activation is helpful during acute infection; however, uncontrolled TH17 activity is associated with autoimmune pathology.[57]] Mycotoxin is an extremely difficult thing to get rid of, and it's rarely recognized by anybody in mainstream medicine because they don't know about labs that test for it. They don't know that they can do a urine test and look for*

---

56 https://www.ncbi.nlm.nih.gov/pubmed/24192494
57 https://www.jci.org/articles/view/78085

these mycotoxins and other pathogens. It's not on their radar, so what they do is if it looks like some of these other really serious brain diseases, they do a couple of scans, they don't see anything, they say, "Well, everything looks fine." Then they make a psych referral. They send them off for some SSRIs (selective serotonin reuptake inhibitors—commonly used to treat depression and other mood disorders).

One needs to begin to rule out some of these things like myco-toxins. The simplest way to do it and the cheapest way to do it is actually to get a test kit, take a little dust from your vacuum cleaner, and you test it. It's really important with anybody, but especially the children, to rule out the mycotoxin element as part of this syndrome because it turns off the immune system for the mycotoxin for its own benefit, so to speak.

Can you speak a little on how you manage PANS in your clinic?

When I take in a new patient I check some reflex points, and I do a lot of muscle testing. I look to see what emotional baggage this person brings to the table. Is it anxiety? Is it fear? These kids are over the top with anxiety. They're over the top with fear, and I try to resolve those emotions. Bach flower remedies are really great to actually downregulate some of the emotions and hyper excitability that you see with these kids. You can put the remedies on the bottom of their feet if they can't take it internally. You can get creams of certain ones; you can just rub it on their ears. You can start with simple things like that.

The next thing that I look at are aggravants, and the aggravants might be an unresolved virus, an unresolved bacteria, an unresolved mold issue.

Viruses are always followed by bacteria, which are always followed by mold, and then it's always followed by detox. So when the body is dealing with each of these, the body needs to find a way to excrete them. The body is really good at handling the virus or the bacteria or the mold. What it's very bad at is excreting that stuff and getting it out of the body. I look for ways to help the body deal with and excrete all of these aggravants,

You talk about aggravants like viruses, bacteria and mold; what about other toxic exposures like pesticides? What role do pesticides play in all of this?

I'm here in Southern California. We have grass all year around. We have green trees all year around, and we have people all year around that are out there spraying it with RoundUp in their white suits in a mask. The lucky ones are doing that. That stuff is just in everything. When I check for aggravants, everybody has a pesticide component, and it's RoundUp.

Let me give you an example of how this impacts us. I'm teaching a patient seminar, and at the beginning of the seminar I show a picture of my two-year old granddaughter towing an empty little red wagon. Then I show my older grandchild with the wagon that has been loaded up with bottles of pesticides and sprays and bad food and pizza. The point is that our exposures are so varied and so nasty that our bodies can't keep up. These pictures of my grandkids towing their little red wagon that are supposed to be empty but instead are full and overflowing with things that they cannot excrete.

Our detoxification pathways can't keep up with this toxic burden. That's why younger and younger people are getting diseases that were traditionally older people's diseases. In the past it took someone 80 years to accumulate the stuff to get prostate cancer. Now we're accumulating these things as children.

How would you advise someone to build resilience so they can better tolerate this toxic burden? What are the best ways for people to build their own resilience?

Well, it's a matter of figuring out how to get these toxins out. They get out by supporting detoxification pathways by eating cruciferous vegetables, sulfur, and supporting the MTHFR variation if they have it. They're getting out through phase one, the glutathione pathway, the sulfation pathway, all the stuff that's part of phase two.

*Doctors should be looking at detoxification pathways. They should be looking at phase-one, phase-two, and phase-three detoxification. [**Editor's Note:** Dr. Watkinson is referring to three phases of detoxification that the liver uses to eliminate toxins from the body.] You have to get toxins out of the cell, and the way you get them out of the cell is you get things into the cell that will cause it to excrete, and that needs to be fat-soluble stuff. Butyric acid is one example. It is a short-chain fatty acid that is reparative in the gut. It can cross the blood-brain barrier. It can get inside the cell. If there are not enough good fats entering the cell (through diet or supplementation) to push that stuff out and then get rid of it, that's another big reason why people cannot detoxify.*

Liposomal glutathione can be helpful. But there's a big, big difference in the liposomal glutathiones. We've had three or four different ones here in the office, and some of them work, and some of them don't. If a physician is not muscle testing many of these products, you'll be using products that can go rancid.

What are your thoughts on biofilms and how they might make it more difficult for the body to eliminate pathogens?

*A lot of people have been chasing biofilms. It's an old conversation. What I've found really makes the difference is to attack it from its calcium meshwork that holds it all together. If you treat that calcium portion of it and degrade the strength of the calcium, the whole biofilm falls apart. [**Editor's Note:** More on calcium and biofilm can be found in the footnote.[58]] What I use to break up biofilm is a Standard Process product, and that actually breaks down that calcium network that holds the biofilm together, and then after that you have to put a lot of good stuff in to get the bad stuff out, but if you start with that phospholipid, it actually will take that matrix apart.*

---

58 http://journals.plos.org/plosone/article?id=10.1371/journal.pone.0091935

What is your opinion on the importance of microbes versus terrain, and how do you feel about antimicrobials as a therapeutic tool?

Many mainstream doctors have been taught a "kill" mentality. We're always looking for new ways to kill the germs--use landmines, bigger bombs, and better technology to find it because we just need to kill it. You use that mentality and you pay a price for it. You're much better off getting the body to clean its own house, to get it to detoxify itself appropriately so that when the thing is killed by either you or anything else, for that matter, when it's killed, it can leave. It can be excreted. The biggest problem with the kill mentality is they put nothing in there to help your body excrete. They use your body as a battleground, and using your body as a battleground is not a fruitful way to restore the health of the individual. They may get over part of it for a little bit and symptoms may change, but really getting it out of them is a bigger issue.

*Now, we've found there are technologies that some physicians use where you can invert the frequency of these causative agents and give them back to people, and in fact that then stops it in its tracks. It goes away, but you've got to support the detoxification of it because what you're doing is giving the body the armament to solve its own problems, to fix its own problems, but if you don't supply the necessary ingredients of getting it out of the body after you did it, you're never going to actually make the ground that you want to make. [**Editor's Note:** Dr. Watkinson is talking about using vibrational therapies that use frequencies as "antimicrobials" rather than pharmaceutical, herbal or other types of antimicrobials].*

What are the basics that you think have to be present in order for the healing process to begin?

Do your best to get away from wireless technology wherever possible. You can paint your house with WiFi blocking paint, you can put film on the windows, you can move someplace where there are none of these aggravants that are going to be affecting your child. You need to make sure that the pathways of excretion in your body are working. You need to be able to have a food chain that you can rely on. The problem with the food chain today is you go to the best of grocery stores, and the food is not fresh.

You've got to have a really good reliable source of food, whether or not you grow it yourself or find a farmer's market that actually can deliver food to you from parts of the country that are not crazed with the use of pesticides and stuff and fish that may come from a good source that comes from Alaska that is not rancid. It's hard to find.

If you live on the West Coast, they used to find the radiation was worse from Fukushima in Oregon and Washington; they're now finding it on the beaches of San Diego. The fish in the West Coast, the tuna, the rest of the fish that come from here, I put on my sheet, my histamine diet, "Don't eat West Coast fish." Just don't eat it. It's got a radiation problem. The thyroid issues that are happening are coming from a progression of binding sites that are being affected by radiation, sticking to these binding sites that are preventing iodine and other nutrients that are sticking to the binding sites because they're being blocked. When you hit bismuth with radiation, it creates something called astatine, and I think that's the guy that's actually binding and preventing, so people get hyperactive and hypoactive thyroid symptoms with a thyroid that's actually being bound with other metals, radioactive metals, that shouldn't be on those binding sites at all.

Then there is the problem of mandated vaccines. That would be my next thing on the list. Healthy food, healthy detox, no vaccines. None, none, none. Zero, zero, zero. That would be the next thing on the list because you need to go through a detox to get rid of what vaccines put in you.

What do you think most frequently causes the opening of the blood-brain barrier in children with PANS?

*Radio frequency. Radio frequency opens the blood brain barrier. The cerebellum is a brain organ, and it is mostly thought of as something that helps you with balance, okay? Well, it not only helps with balance, but it's very connected to the whole immune system in your body, which is the hypothalamus, so when you get a concussion, what happens is part of that is affecting the cerebellum, which is then affecting the hypothalamus, which then alters your body's ability to fight infections because what happens to you at that point is you upregulate TH17, you downregulate T1 and T2 [**Editor's Note:** Here Dr. Toby is referring to the upregulation of TH17 cells, again, associated with autoimmunity, and the downregulation of TH1 and TH2 cells, which would otherwise bring balance back to the immune response].*

What kind of fats do you recommend for people to eat?

*Well, I think the one item that really has made a major difference with a lot of kids is the whole Bravo yogurt movement. [**Editor's Note:** Bravo yogurt is a probiotic food made from fermented milk; the starter culture contains dozens of probiotic strains of bacteria and yeast]. I think the Bravo yogurt is an excellent addition for getting the immune system straightened back out. I would start there with a lot of the kids. It can help to get their gut and brain on the same page with something like a Bravo yogurt.*

GLOSSARY

Acupressure

In this type of therapy, pressure is applied to the body with fingers to the same points used in acupuncture *(see listing)*. It is used for the relief of pain, tension or energy blocks.

Acupuncture

This form of Traditional Chinese Medicine has been practiced for centuries to release blocks or imbalances in "chi," the body's energy that flows through and around the body along pathways called meridians *(see listing)*. Despite the fact that fine needles are inserted into the skin along meridians, it is typically painless and is often relaxing. Acupuncturists may use tools other than needles when treating children.

Allergy

Allergy refers to both immediate (IgE) and delayed reactions (IgA). A true allergy is a specific immediate reaction such as hives, congestion or swelling involving an antibody called Immunoglobulin E (IgE; *see listing*). Traditional scratch testing is used to identify IgE triggers, such as pollen, peanuts, or strawberries that can cause symptoms ranging from annoying to lethal. People with an IgE allergy may need to carry injectable epinephrine to treat life-threatening anaphylaxis that can lead to a drop in blood pressure and difficulty breathing. Most allergists test only for IgE allergies and do not test for sensitivities and intolerances *(see listing)* that are known as IgA *(see listing)*, IgG *(see listing)* and IgM *(see listing)*.

Allopathic Medicine (Western Medicine)

Allopathic, or Western, Medicine describes a practice of medicine wherein physicians treat disease through the use of drugs or surgery. The term allopathic is often used with negative connotations when referring to the practice of suppressing symptoms with pharmaceuticals, rather than searching out and treating root causes of disease such as gut dysbiosis *(see listing)*, immune dysregulation *(see listing)*, toxicity, inflammation, nutritional deficiencies *(see listing)* or hormonal imbalances. Most pharmaceutical medications create side effects, nutritional deficiencies and toxicity. In the case of children with PANS, the typical allopathic approach is to treat it with antibiotics *(see listing)*, IVIG *(see listing)* and/or plasmapharesis *(see listing)*.

Anat Baniel Method

By accessing the powers of neuroplasticity and the brain's ability to change itself, this method of bodywork helps people discover how to improve the mind and body dramatically enhancing physical, cognitive, emotional and creative performance. The Anat Baniel method builds upon the work of Dr. Moshe Feldenkrais.

Anorexia

This type of eating disorder can be a symptom that is triggered by infection such as PANS. Children with this disorder may restrict the amount and/or types of food eaten, causing weight loss or lack appropriate weight gain. In children with PANS, food restriction may be due more to a food phobia rather than an unhealthy body image. If food restriction is of sudden-onset, work with your child's healthcare practitioner to screen for PANS.

Antibiotic

This type of antimicrobial drug, commonly produced by or synthesized from molds, is used in the treatment of bacterial infection. The most commonly used antibiotics to fight the bacteria associated with PANS and PANDAS infections are penicillin, amoxicillin (including Augmentin) and cephalosporins. Erythromycin, azithromycin and clindamycin are also commonly used. *Note: Antibiotic resistance is common, so their use should be judicious.*

Antibody

Antibodies are immunoglobulins *(see listing)* produced by the immune system in response to the presence of toxins or foreign pathogens in the body called antigens. Antibodies contain specific binding sites that recognize and neutralize antigens.

Anti-NMDA Receptor Encephalitis

This type of autoimmune disorder wherein the body produces antibodies that attack NMDA (N-methyl-D-aspartate)-type glutamate receptors in the brain causes inflammation and a variety of symptoms including headache, seizures and psychosis. It was brought to the public's attention with Susannah Cahalan's 2013 book, *Brain on Fire: My Month of Madness.* It is essentially an adult form of PANS. *(See listings for Glutamate, NMDA and Psychosis.)*

Anti-Streptococcal DNase B

This is one of several blood tests used to identify post-streptococcal infections by assessing the presence of antibodies specific to Group A *Streptococcus.* The presence of these antibodies is not a conclusive diagnosis of PANS, as it is a clinical diagnosis.

Anti-Streptolysin O (ASO)

This is a blood titer that detects the presence of antibodies to Group A *Streptococcus* and is a means of assessing recent or acute streptococcal infection. The presence of these antibodies is not a conclusive diagnosis of PANS, as it is a clinical diagnosis.

Anxiety

Anxiety is characterized as the body's physical reaction to real or perceived fear, stress, or danger as a sense of panic, uneasiness, distress, or dread. Anxiety disorders can keep people from sleeping, concentrating, talking to others, or even leaving their home. Anxiety that may need treatment is often irrational, overwhelming, and disproportionate to the situation. It makes sufferers feel as though they have no control of their feelings, and it can involve serious physical symptoms like headaches, nausea, or trembling. When normal anxiety becomes irrational and begins to recur and interfere with daily life, it is classified as a disorder. Western medicine is beginning to understand that anxiety may have a physiological basis such as a magnesium deficiency, lithium orotate deficiency, GABA deficiency, retained Moro reflex *(see Primitive Reflexes)* and/or an infection that crosses the blood-brain barrier such as PANS. Children in a state of anxiety are in a state of sympathetic nervous system *(see listing)* dominance, also known as "fight or flight."

Applied Kinesiology

This type of assessment tool is not a replacement for conventional medical testing but can be used as an additional form of testing. Its premise is based on the theory that everything, including the body, is made up of energy and that the body responds to energy from other things in either a positive or negative way. Things or thoughts that may be harmful to the body are experienced as weakness in the muscles, which is why this form of testing is also called "muscle testing." Applied kinesiology may be especially helpful in working with children, as it is non-invasive.

Attention Deficit Disorders (ADD/ADHD)

This is a neurodevelopmental disorder *(see listing)* defined by specific subjective criteria such as poor concentration, lack of focus, easy frustration, explosive anger and low self-esteem. A child with symptoms of hyperactivity and impulsive behavior in addition to the above criteria may be identified as having Attention Deficit Hyperactivity Disorder (ADHD). There is no blood test for ADD/ADHD, and the diagnosis is determined by observation of behaviors in at least two settings. Western medicine is beginning to understand that ADD/ADHD may be related to anomalies in the gut microbiome *(see listing)*, immune dysregulation *(see listing)*, nutritional deficiencies *(see listing)*, vision processing *(see listing for Vision)*, auditory processing, sensory processing *(see listing)*, retained primitive reflexes *(see listing)*, neurotransmitter imbalances (especially dopamine *(see listing)*), food sensitivities/intolerances *(see listing)*, and environmental toxins such as lead, fluoride and BPA. More knowledgeable practitioners now believe that a large percentage of children with ADD/ADHD may also have PANS. Children can lose their diagnosis of ADD/ADHD by addressing the root causes of toxicity, gut dysbiosis *(see listing)*, immune dysregulation *(see listing)*, nutritional deficiencies, genetic mutations *(see listing)*, hormonal imbalances and inflammation while implementing therapies that rewire the brain and central nervous system.

Auditory Integration Therapy (AIT)

Drs. Guy Berard and Alfred Tomatis developed this type of auditory therapy in France as a way to retrain the brain to help normalize hearing, senses and brain processing. AIT can improve a child's language, focus, concentration, cognitive skills and communication skills. More importantly, it can reduce sensitivities to sound, meltdowns, aggressive behaviors and hyperactivity, which can be common symptoms in children with PANS. A child who undergoes this type of therapy will likely be tested beforehand to determine which sound-frequency ranges he or she is over- or undersensitive. A therapeutic plan typically entails two sessions per day for a length of 30 minutes each for 10 consecutive days. During a session, the child will listen to pre-selected music or sounds that can balance over- or under-sensitivity to sound-frequency ranges.

Autism Spectrum Disorder (ASD)

ASD is a neurodevelopmental disorder *(see listing)* characterized by impairments in sensory, language, social-emotional and behavior areas. It is a "spectrum disorder," with manifestations ranging from mild to severe, depending on the level of social impairment, communication impairment and restricted, repetitive patterns of behavior. Children with severe ASD may exhibit self-stimulating behavior ("stimming") such as rocking or hand flapping. Because children with ASD often have obsessive thoughts and compulsive behaviors, more knowledgeable practitioners now believe that a large percentage of children with ASD may also have PANS. Western medicine is beginning to understand that ASD may be related to anomalies in nutrient levels, the gut microbiome *(see listing)*, immune dysregulation *(see listing)*, vision processing *(see listing for Vision)*, auditory processing, sensory processing *(see listing)*, retained primitive reflexes *(see listing)*, neurotransmitter imbalances *(see listing)*, food sensitivities/intolerances *(see listing)*, excitotoxins *(see listing)*, and environmental toxins such as mercury. Children can lose their diagnosis of autism by addressing these root causes while implementing therapies that rewire the brain and central nervous system.

Autoimmune Disorder/Disease

This is an inflammatory condition in which antibodies, which are protein molecules produced by the body's immune system, are believed to attack and destroy healthy body tissue. Recent research is beginning to point out that the body may not be attacking itself, however, as previously thought. Instead, the body may be attacking infectious agents such as herpetic viruses that may currently be evading testing. Women are three times more likely than men to develop an autoimmune disease/disorder. Common examples are PANS, rheumatoid arthritis, celiac disease, Type 1 diabetes, Crohn's disease, psoriasis, lupus and scleroderma.

Autoimmune Encephalitis

This type of swelling of the brain is a serious medical condition in which the immune system mistakenly attacks the brain, leading to inflammation and impaired function. It can result from infections such as PANS, but not all causes are known. Psychiatric manifestations and memory loss are common early in the course of autoimmune encephalitis. Motor symptoms (especially in children) and seizures may also be present.

Basal Ganglia

The basal ganglia are a group of nuclei linked to the thalamus that are located at the base of the brain that facilitate movement and inhibit competing movements, which is why they have traditionally been associated with movement disorders, such as Huntington's and Parkinson's disease. In addition to voluntary movement control, the basal ganglia are also associated with procedural learning *(see listing)*, eye movements, cognitive function and emotional function. The basal ganglia are the site of two dopamine *(see listing)* receptors. In PANS, the cross-reactive antibodies *(see listing)* created in response to an infection attack the dopamine receptors in the basal ganglia of the brain because of a blood-brain barrier *(see listing)* breach.

B Cells

B lymphocytes, known as "B cells," are a type of small, white blood cell that does some of the work of the immune system. They mature in the bone and are the equivalent of pedestrians jumping up and down outside a burning building yelling, "FIRE! FIRE!" The B cell's job is to "draw attention to the burning building." In immune disorders such as PANS, there is an over-proliferation of B cells and not enough T cells *(see listing)* that can organize and stop the cause of the immune-system attack.

Bioenergetic Medicine

This type of energy medicine medicine is founded on the idea that the body is a flow system. All particles have charge and are therefore interacting in positive and negative ways. As such, understanding the interaction of molecular frequencies is vital to understanding the innate workings of the body.

Biofeedback

Biofeedback is a non-invasive technique using electrical sensors that measure and give information (feedback) about the body (bio). By using biofeedback, a child can learn to control the body's functions, such as breathing, heart rate and skin temperature. By focusing on the feedback, a child can learn to make subtle changes in the body, such as relaxing certain muscles, and learn to reduce pain, anxiety *(see listing)* and stress.

Biomedical Protocol

This type of medicine is synonymous with functional medicine *(see listing)*, which aims to identify root causes of diseases and disorders rather than treating symptoms with just pharmaceuticals. Typically, there is more than one root cause underlying a condition, and people with a chronic condition often have root causes such as nutritional deficiencies *(see listing)*, gut dysbiosis *(see listing)*, immune dysregulation *(see listing)*, hormonal imbalances, metabolic imbalances, toxicity and inflammation. Children with PANS, as well as those with neurodevelopmental disorders *(see listing)*, asthma, allergies and autoimmune conditions often benefit from a biomedical protocol.

Biomeridian Testing

The Biomeridian is an electroacupuncture *(see listing)* machine that assesses the energy flow along specific meridians *(see listing)* in the body to determine the relative strength or weakness of an organ or system.

BioRegulation Therapy (BRT)

This type of therapy uses a combination of biofeedback *(see listing)* and PEMF-based *(see listing)* electromagnetic technology to help the body better self-regulate, adapt and heal naturally. BRT amplifies the "healthy" harmonic frequencies and sends them back to the cells to help the nervous system calm down. The body's nervous system then uses that feedback to reorganize itself and improve its own intercellular communication. With the feedback, the cells better align themselves within the organ system and entire body. BRT can promote a sense of relaxation and calm, which is helpful for the anxiety *(see listing)* that most children with PANS have.

BioSET

Bio-Energetic Sensitivity and Enzyme Therapy, also known as BioSET, is used to lower the body's immune response to ordinarily benign substances such as food, dander and pollen. It was developed by Ellen Culter, DC and uses techniques and philosophies of functional medicine *(see listing)*, homeopathy *(see listing)*, acupressure *(see listing)*, acupuncture *(see listing)*, applied kinesiology *(see listing)*, chiropractic care *(see listing)*, Traditional Chinese Medicine, enzyme therapy, craniosacral therapy *(see listing)*, applied immunology, and integrative medicine nutrition.

Blomberg Rhythmic Movement Training

This type of motor training program, known as RMT, was developed by Dr. Harald Blomberg and is used to improve motor abilities and motor control such as muscle tone, coordination, and integration of primitive reflexes *(see listing)*. Other areas of dysfunction such as vision *(see listing)*, speech, attention, hyperactivity, writing and reading and may also improve with these movements. It is especially helpful for children with neurodevelopmental disorders *(see listing)* but can also be used to decrease anxiety *(see listing)* that children with PANS typically have.

Blood-Brain Barrier

This protective network of blood vessels can keep certain things like toxins and pathogens out of the brain. Importantly, the blood-brain barrier also keeps out antibodies *(see listing)*. In PANS, however, a breach to the blood-brain barrier allows antibodies into the brain. If the antibodies are targeting brain tissues, receptors and cells, then this breakdown of the barrier is problematic. This allows the immune system to actually start attacking the brain itself. Recent research has shown that a number of things can cause a blood-brain-barrier breach such as antibiotics *(see listing)*, Traumatic Brain Injury or concussion, ElectroMagnetic Fields *(see listing)*, toxins from injectable adjuvants, stress, trauma, chemical exposure, toxin exposure, ultrasounds, wheat *(see listing for Gluten)* and infections from viruses, bacteria and fungi.

Body Ecology Diet (BED)

The Body Ecology Diet, developed by Donna Gates, is a gut-healing diet that can eliminate gut dysbiosis *(see listing)*, correct nutritional deficiencies *(see listing)*, strengthen the adrenal glands, and conquer systemic infections. A healthy gut produces nutrients for the brain, and a healthy liver *(see listing)* removes toxins from the body. Western medicine is beginning to understand that the health of the brain is very much dependent on the health of the gut, which is why the gut is called "the second brain." The Body Ecology Diet is based on the principles of contraction/expansion, acid/alkaline, individualization, food combining, the 80/20 principle, cleansing and the step-by-step principle.

Candida

Although *Candida* is a common yeast-like fungus in most people, it can overgrow in a child with gut dysbiosis *(see listing)*, leading to symptoms such as acid reflux, constipation, diarrhea, thrush and vaginal yeast infections. Because the gastrointestinal system is the most common site of *Candida* overgrowth and because the gastrointestinal system houses about 50-70% of the body's immune system, a *Candida* overgrowth can also contribute to asthma, allergies, mood disorders, neurodevelopmental disorders *(see listing)*, PANS and autoimmune disorders *(see listing)*. Common causes of *Candida* overgrowth are usage of antibiotics (both maternally and for the child; *see listing*), Motrin, Advil, ibuprofen, C-section birth, a Standard American Diet *(see listing)*, and antibiotic-containing foods such as non-organic meats, dairy and seafood as well as crops grown with glyphosate, found in the RoundUp weed killer.

Casein

This protein found in mammalian milk is a common cause of food intolerance/sensitivity *(see listing)*. Casein intolerance is not the same thing as lactose intolerance, as casein is a protein, and lactose is a sugar. Children with PANS often have a casein intolerance/sensitivity and can benefit from the removal of it from their diet. Doing so can lower the total load of stressors, including chronic inflammation, on the body's immune system. Casein is found in all animal milk products, such as cheese, milk, yogurt and ice cream, but the casein found in camel's milk is of a different structure and is typically better tolerated. In addition, digestive enzymes and allergy elimination techniques such as BioSET *(see listing)* can lower the immune system's sensitivity to casein.

Childhood Acute Neuropsychiatric Symptoms (CANS)

This terminology refers to a syndrome that is similar to PANS, but it downplays the role of *Strep* or other infections. Coined by Howard Singer MD, it requires only the acute, dramatic onset of symptoms.

Chiropractor

This type of healthcare provider specializes in nervous-system and musculoskeletal system issues and aims to correct these issues by manually adjusting the body's structure. Doctors of Chiropractic (DC) are not licensed to prescribe medication. Children with PANS often have misalignments in the cranial, upper cervical and pelvic areas caused by birth trauma, injury or other trauma that can weaken the brain's and body's ability to protect itself; chiropractors can adjust these misalignments. Chiropractors may also typically provide information about dietary and lifestyle changes as well as therapies and exercises that can improve and maintain health.

Cognitive Behavioral Therapy (CBT)

Cognitive Behavioral Therapy is a type of psychotherapy that works on changing one's thoughts and ultimately behaviors. The goal of CBT is to change thought patterns or beliefs (distorted or valid), attitudes, and ultimately behavior to help a child face challenges and more effectively work toward goals. Children with PANS can benefit from CBT.

Convergence Disorder

This eye-teaming problem is a common vision *(see listing)* problem in children with PANS as well as those with neurodevelopmental disorders *(see listing)*, perhaps because many children with neurodevelopmental disorders also have PANS. In convergence disorder, the eyes tend to drift outward when a child is reading or doing close work, leading to double vision. To prevent seeing double, a child may try to make the eyes turn back in (converge), which then interferes with the ability to read and work comfortably at near distances. A convergence disorder can be corrected with vision therapy prescribed by a developmental optometrist *(see listing)*.

Craniosacral Therapy (CST)

This type of bodywork therapy is a very gentle, relaxing and hands-on intervention that can help with many physical and emotional issues. CST aims to enhance the balanced motion of the membrane layers surrounding the brain (the meninges), blood and cerebrospinal fluid moving into and out of the cranium as well as areas of the body that might be straining the craniosacral system and the brain. CST often brings about a profound sense of peace and relaxation. Many parents report that children who undergo CST often sleep better and are less prone to outbursts and anxiety.

Cunningham Panel

This is a series of tests that was developed by Madeleine Cunningham, PhD to help physicians diagnose and treat infection-induced neuropsychiatric disorders. These tests measure circulating levels of auto-antibodies directed against specific neuronal antigens, including dopamine *(see listing)* D1 receptor (DRD1), dopamine D2L receptor (DRD2L), lysoganglioside GM1 *(see listing)* and tubulin *(see listing)*. According to Moleculera Labs, "The purpose of the Cunningham Panel is to provide laboratory results that assist physicians in diagnosing infection-induced autoimmune neuropsychiatric disorders." A positive Cunningham Panel is often used to confirm that a child has an autoimmune disease *(see listing)* affecting the brain. For many doctors and families, the Cunningham Panel has been used to convince naysayers that there is a serious medical condition present and not just some "psychiatric" problem that can be treated with psychotropic medications or cognitive behavioral therapy. This test is used as a diagnostic tool for PANS but is not required for clinical diagnosis.

Depression

Children with PANS often report being in a state of depression, which is a prolonged state of sadness and unhappiness or mood dysregulation. Somatic expression *(see listing)* of these persistent feelings can result in poor concentration, lack of energy and an inability to sleep well. In some cases, PANS children with depression may have suicidal tendencies or rage.

Developmental Optometrist

This type of eye doctor (OD) is educated in the behavioral and functional aspects of vision *(see listing)*, which is not the same thing as eyesight (acuity). Eyesight is the sharpness of the image seen by the eye; vision is the brain's ability to focus on and comprehend that which is seen. Vision processing problems are common in children with PANS as well as neurodevelopmental disorders *(see listing)*, motor delays and vestibular difficulties. A developmental optometrist, also known as a behavioral optometrist, often uses lenses, prisms and vision therapy to enhance and improve visual function. These interventions can improve a child's academic and behavioral stamina as well as the ability to focus.

Dialectical Behavior Therapy (DBT)

This type of psychotherapy combines cognitive and behavioral therapies. The goal of DBT is to identify and change negative-thinking patterns and destructive behaviors into positive outcomes. DBT skills include skills for mindfulness, emotion regulation, distress tolerance, and interpersonal effectiveness. DBT can be helpful for children with PANS.

Dirty Electricity

This type of ElectroMagnetic Field *(see listing)* comes from off-phase electrical systems and wiring in houses and buildings. It can be rectified by plugging in Stetzer filters into electrical outlets at set intervals.

DNaseB

This protein is produced by Group A *Streptococcus*, and the body makes antibodies *(see listing)* to these proteins. The blood test to look for these antibodies is called Anti-DNase B *(see listing)*. More than 90% of past streptococcal infections can be correctly identified with the combination of the Anti-DNase B and the Anti-Strep-tolysin O (ASO) blood test *(see listing)*.

Dopamine

This molecule is both a pleasure-producing neurotransmitter *(see listing)* and hormone *(see listing)*, making it a member of the cat-echolamine class of molecules. It is important for feelings of hap-piness, motor movement and cognition. Low dopamine affects the ability to focus and think, while high dopamine causes an overload on the brain's ability to process information. According to the mo-lecular mimicry *(see listing)* theory, when the cross-reactive anti-bodies *(see listing)* associated with *Strep* or other antigens associ-ated with PANS attack the dopamine receptors in the basal ganglia of the brain, it causes a fluctuation in dopamine, which results in OCD *(see listing)*, tics *(see listing)* and other neuropsychiatric symptoms. Some doctors also refer to this as autoimmune-medi-ated basal ganglia *(see listing)* dysfunction.

Dyslexia

This type of neurodevelopmental disorder *(see listing)* is marked by a severe difficulty in the brain's ability to process the smallest sounds of language, phonemes, which in turn makes it difficult to map sounds to letters. This can lead to problems with reading, writ-ing and spelling at grade level. Although these children are often bright, their disability often leads to them having low self-esteem. Dyslexia can be improved by addressing the root causes of toxic-ity, gut dysbiosis *(see listing)*, immune dysregulation *(see listing)*, nutritional deficiencies *(see listing)*, hormonal imbalances and in-flammation while implementing therapies that rewire the brain and central nervous system. Research supports using an Orton-Gilling-ham approach to reading, which is a phonetic, structured, sequen-tial and multisensory approach to reading. Children with dyslexia often respond very well to vision therapy *(see listing for Vision)*.

Eczema (Atopic Dermatitis)

This type of inflammatory skin condition is characterized by red, itchy skin and the formation of scaly or crusty patches on the skin that may leak fluid or pus. Eczema is a common condition in babies and toddlers that often stems from the use of antibiotics *(see listing)* maternally, during birth, or by the child. Antibiotics disrupt the gut microbiome *(see listing)*, which in turn disrupts the immune system *(see listing for Immune Dysregulation)*. Children with PANS are more likely to have or have had eczema, as it is a soft sign of a dysregulated immune system. Western medicine typically addresses eczema with topical steroids such as cortisone cream, but this can lead to steroid dependence and often drives the disease process deeper into the body, potentially leading to asthma. Because the skin is the body's largest organ of detoxification, eczema is typically a sign that other organs of elimination such as the liver *(see listing)*, kidneys, lungs and gut are congested. Because naturopathic doctors *(see listing)* are educated about the body's detoxification organs, lymphatic drainage systems and the effect that dietary changes can have on health, they are often a good choice of practitioner for help with this condition.

Electroacupuncture

This type of acupuncture *(see listing)* uses a small electric current passed between pairs of acupuncture needles. It can be used to increase the effectiveness of regular acupuncture for symptoms such as pain and anxiety *(see listing)*.

ElectroDermal Screening (EDS)

This type of painless, non-invasive assessment tool was originally known as Electroacupuncture According to Voll (EAV), after its inventor, Dr. Reinhard Voll, a German medical doctor and engineer. It measures the electrical conductance of the skin to the passage of a small, unfelt electrical current and uses the same principle used for lie detectors and biofeedback devices *(see listing)*. These assessment devices are typically bundled with software that is programmed to read imbalances in bodily systems. They do not diagnose medical conditions; rather, they are used to support a clinician's assessment. ASYRA and Zyto *(see listing)* are some of the brand names of these devices.

ElectroMagnetic Fields (EMFs)

Scientists have known since the 1830's that electrical fields are also magnetic, a concept discovered by Michael Faraday and known as electromagnetism. Today's electrical devices, especially wireless ones, give off far-greater and more-dangerous levels of these electromagnetic waves known as EMFs. Devices such as cell phones, cordless house phones, baby monitors, Wi-Fi systems and smart meters give off strong levels of EMFs, while fluorescent lights, hairdryers, fans and large electrical devices such as TVs, stoves and refrigerators do as well. Research shows that EMFs can cause changes in both the sympathetic nervous system *(see listing)* as well as the parasympathetic nervous system *(see listing)*, leading to symptoms such as heart palpitations, memory problems, difficulty concentrating, sleep problems, headaches, feeling unwell, dizziness, tinnitus and chronic fatigue. Children with PANS often benefit from the removal of EMFs and the avoidance of EMFs in public spaces such as schools.

Emotional Freedom Technique (EFT)/Tapping

This bodywork tool, also known as tapping, can be used to relieve stress and anxiety *(see listing)* while improving emotional, physical and performance issues. By tapping with the fingertips on certain acupressure points on the head and upper body while making positive statements about a situation, a sense of well-being and release can be achieved. Children can typically learn to do this technique for themselves very easily, and children with PANS, as well as their parents, can benefit from this technique for self-care.

Encephalitis

Inflammation and swelling of the brain can be caused by an infection that crosses the blood-brain barrier *(see listing)*, such as in PANS, as well as from toxic assault, allergic reaction, concussion or other type of brain injury. Encephalitis is increasingly common in children and babies today, as the number of children with PANS, seizures, autism *(see listing)* and other neurological disorders continues to increase. An increase in a child's head-circumference percentile, especially in the first year of life, can signal encephalitis to an astute clinician.

Essential Oils

These concentrated oils from plants have many medicinal properties in addition to their pleasing odors. They can be inhaled, used topically or ingested, depending on the type of oil. Not only can they be used to replace common toxic household and personal-care products, but they can also be used to promote health. Certain essential oils such as frankincense, oregano, cinnamon, clove, tea tree and copaiba are used by parents for their children with PANS to boost their immune systems.

Excitotoxicity

This is the process by which nerve cells are damaged or killed by excessive stimulation by neurotransmitters such as glutamate *(see listing)*. Excitotoxicity can cause encephalitis *(see listing)* and seizures. The N-methyl-D-aspartate receptor (also known as the NMDA receptor, *see listing*) is a glutamate receptor found in nerve cells that is activated when the amino acids glutamate and glycine bind to it. NMDA receptors have been implicated by a number of studies to be strongly involved with excitotoxicity.

Exposure Therapy

Exposure Therapy is a type of Cognitive Behavioral Therapy *(see listing)*. With Response and Prevention Therapy (E/RP), the person is exposed to a trigger and learns how to be uncomfortable to the point where he or she can ignore the trigger. With E/RP, a therapist exposes the person to situations that trigger his or her obsessions and compulsions. The emphasis is on learning how to deal with the uncomfortableness rather than avoid it, as the latter leads to negative reinforcement. Over time, through exposures, psycho-education, and Cognitive Behavioral Therapy, the person learns to respond differently to these triggers, leading to a decrease in the frequency of compulsions and the intensity of obsessions. Exposure Therapy can be helpful to a child with PANS.

Eye Movement Desensitization and Reprocessing (EMDR)

EMDR is a powerful psychotherapy technique developed by Francine Shapiro, PhD. It is very successful in helping people who suffer from trauma, anxiety *(see listing)*, panic, disturbing memories, post-traumatic stress *(see listing for PTSD)* and many other emotional problems. Tactile, audio and visual stimulation is used to activate the opposite sides of the brain to help release emotional experiences that are "trapped" in the nervous system. It is based on the premise that "whatever fires together wires together." Therefore, the goal is to reprocess the trauma and allow the "rational brain" to kick in to free the "emotional brain" of the high levels of emotion tied to the trauma to achieve a more peaceful state. EMDR can be helpful to a child with PANS.

Family Constellations Therapy

Developed by Dr. Bert Hellinger, renowned German psychoanalyst, family constellations therapy is a very powerful type of energy medicine tool for healing multi-generational psychological wounds such as trauma, dysfunctional relationships, loss, abuse and family drama. Dr. Hellinger believed that dysfunction, suffering and unhappiness often relate to painful events in a family's past, instead of originating in a person's current life history. Dietrich Klinghardt, MD, PhD, believes that children with chronic illnesses such as autism *(see listing)*, other neurodevelopmental disorders *(see listing)* and PANS are particularly vulnerable to disturbances in the family's energy field. Unhealed trans-generational family issues create a disturbance in the field, which filters down into a child's psyche, nervous system, and metabolic functioning. Family constellations usually take place in a group moderated by a facilitator, and an individual with a concern chooses representatives for members of his/her family from the group. The individual then positions these representatives in a way that feels right and then watches as they may begin to experience physical sensations, emotions, or urges belonging not to themselves, but to the family members they represent, known as the "knowing field." Through observations, questions, trial statements, and movements, the facilitator and individual may come to see the issue in a new way, potentially leading to a resolution that enables the client to break his/her connection with difficulties in the family's past.

Food Sensitivity/Intolerance

This type of immune response often involves a delayed onset of symptoms to foods, chemical preservatives, toxicity and/or a variety of pathogens which can take up to several hours, or even days, to appear. These often go undiagnosed or misdiagnosed because delayed reactions can be hard to detect. They are characterized by an inflammatory response that is not detectable with a typical IgE *(see listing)* test (the test used to diagnose "true allergies"), thus many physicians overlook these types of IgA *(see listing)*, IgG *(see listing)*, and IgM *(see listing)* immune responses. Symptoms may include abdominal pain, headache, constipation, diarrhea, rashes, irritability, runny nose, stuffy nose and an inability to concentrate. Scientists are now linking food and environmental sensitivities to a variety of chronic health conditions. Gluten *(see listing)*, in particular, has been identified as a common food sensitivity that can contribute to a whole host of chronic inflammatory conditions. Other common food sensitivities/intolerances seen in affected children are eggs, dairy, corn, soy, fish, shellfish, peanuts, tree nuts, citrus and chocolate. An elimination followed by a re-introduction (challenge) of certain of these foods for a period of time can be helpful in reducing immune and behavioral symptoms in children with PANS and other chronic conditions.

Functional Medicine

This newer type of Western medicine addresses the whole person while incorporating his or her complex health and medical history. Rather than relying on pharmaceutical medication to reduce symptoms, a functional-medicine practitioner aims to discover the root causes of a person's chronic health condition such as gut dysbiosis *(see listing)*, immune dysregulation *(see listing)*, inflammation, hormonal imbalances, food sensitivities/intolerances *(see listing)*, and environmental toxins. Functional-medicine practitioners typically find that there is no one root cause of chronic conditions; rather, there is usually a host of factors that contributes to a person's total load of stressors. Because of this, there is usually not just one supplement, lifestyle change or dietary intervention that leads to improvement in symptoms. Children with PANS often benefit from the personalization of this multi-factorial, functional-medicine approach.

GABA (Gamma-AminoButyric Acid)

GABA is an inhibitory amino acid that can counter the excitatory effects of excess glutamate *(see listing)*. It is calming and can improve the body's response to stress, thus lowering symptoms of anxiety *(see listing)* and improving the ability to learn. Children with PANS often benefit from supplementing with GABA.

GAD65 Genetic Mutation

Glutamic acid decarboxylase (GAD) is an enzyme that removes carbon dioxide from glutamate *(see listing)* to convert it into GABA *(see listing)* using the active version of vitamin B_6 known as pyridoxal phosphate. Children with PANS, anxiety *(see listing)*, mood disorders, behavior disorders and neurodevelopmental disorders *(see listing)* often have a mutation *(see listing)* of the GAD65 gene needed to produce this enzyme, and these children often benefit from the supplementation of both pyridoxal phosphate and GABA.

Genetic Mutation

Sometimes referred to as "SNPs" (Single-Nucleotide Polymorphisms), these changes or alterations in the DNA sequence can potentially lead to poor health, disease or even eventual death. Although these mutations can be inherited by one or both parents, it is recently coming to light that exposure to environmental toxins such as radiation, heavy metals, carcinogens and endocrine disruptors may be playing a larger role in the increase in children's chronic health conditions, including PANS. Depending on the type of mutation, necessary chemical reactions in the body are prevented from happening such as the production of enzymes, intra-cell nutrient transport and appropriate utilization of nutrients. The MTHFR genetic defect *(see listing)* is common in children with PANS.

Genetically Modified Organism (GMO)

Genetically modifying an organism involves cutting genes out from one organism and inserting them into another. Although scientists can pinpoint what they want to extract, placing that gene into the DNA of another organism is completely random. Scientists do not yet fully understand living systems thoroughly enough to perform this modification without creating mutations that could be harmful to the environment and our health. Currently, there is no data on the long-term safety of GMOs, although there are numerous reports of adverse reactions from the ingestion of these foods such as allergies, intestinal damage, infertility and even infant mortality. These days, 60-70% of processed foods contain genetically engineered ingredients. The most common sources of GMO foods are soybeans, corn, sugar beets, cottonseed and canola oil. The danger in these crops lies not only in their GMO composition, but also in the fact that they have been genetically modified to withstand much-higher applications of the pesticide RoundUp. Although Monsanto (now owned by Bayer), the company that makes and sells RoundUp, had declared it to be safe for decades, in April 2018 a jury awarded $289 million to a former school groundskeeper because it determined that RoundUp caused his terminal cancer. Avoiding foods containing genetically modified organisms is an important step towards getting healthy. Most dairy and beef from cows injected with the genetically engineered hormone rBGH/rBST or fed genetically modified grains are also a significant source of GMO consumption. Products labeled 100% organic do not contain GMOs under current law. If the label does not say 100% organic, it can contain up to 30% GMOs. Children with PANS often have fewer symptoms when eating a non-GMO diet.

Glutamate

Glutamate is an excitatory neurotransmitter and amino acid that has been implicated by a number of studies to be strongly involved with excitotoxicity *(see listing)*. Although glutamate is necessary for learning and memory, an excess of glutamate can lead to excitotoxicity. Glutamate and its analogs are found in processed foods not only as MSG (monosodium glutamate) but also in chemical food additives such as natural flavoring, artificial flavoring, bouillon, hydrolyzed vegetable protein, soy protein isolate, yeast extract, gelatin, barley malt and soy sauce as well as natural foods such as tomatoes, bone broth and seaweed. Both low blood sugar and a *Strep* infection that has crossed the blood-brain barrier *(see listing for PANDAS)* can also increase glutamate levels in the brain. Children with PANS often benefit from the removal of excess glutamate in the diet and from managing blood-sugar levels.

Glutathione (GSH)

Glutathione is a peptide composed of three amino acids: cysteine, glycine and glutamic acid. It is in a class of molecules called antioxidants, whose primary job is to alleviate oxidative stress *(see listing)*. To detoxify mercury, arsenic, lead, cadmium, and other toxins, GSH provides a thiol group that binds to metals and other poisons; the body then excretes a metal-cysteine mixture. If there is not enough glutathione (or other antioxidant), heavy metals and toxins are stored in fat tissue. The brain, nervous system, breasts and prostate are mostly fat, and therefore become receptacles for environmental poisons. Children with PANS often have low levels of glutathione; thus, they typically have higher levels of toxicity.

Gluten

Gluten is a protein found in wheat, barley, rye and non-gluten-free oats. It can cause an inflammatory response and is a common cause of food sensitivities and intolerances *(see listing)*. Because it is inflammatory, it can lead to damage in the small intestine and an impaired ability to absorb nutrients, even in non-celiac disease patients. Some researchers believe that some of the damage may come from glyphosate, an active ingredient in the RoundUp pesticide. RoundUp is sprayed on wheat at the end of the harvest process to act as a desiccant. The glyphosate within it is also a patented antibiotic and thus can contribute to gut dysbiosis *(see listing)*. Consumption of gluten can contribute to symptoms such as constipation, diarrhea, breathing difficulties, chronic sinus infections, chronic colds, lack of focus, dark circles under the eyes and headaches. In addition, gluten can deactivate the enzyme that converts glutamate *(see listing)* to GABA *(see listing)*. Children with PANS often have fewer physiological and behavioral symptoms while removing it from their diet.

Gluten-Free/Casein-Free Diet (GFCF)

The gluten-free/casein-free diet can help children with PANS *(see listing)*, autism *(see listing)*, ADHD *(see listing)*, Sensory Processing Disorder *(see listing)* as well as those with asthma, allergies, autoimmune disorders *(see listing)* and mood disorders improve their symptoms. Gluten *(see listing)* is a protein found in wheat, barley, rye and non-gluten-free oats, while casein *(see listing)* is a protein found in milk products, such as yogurt, ice cream and cheese, from any animal. Both of these proteins can cause inflammatory responses and are common causes of food sensitivities/intolerances *(see listing)*. Consumption of them can contribute to symptoms such as constipation, diarrhea, breathing difficulties, chronic sinus infections, chronic colds, lack of focus, dark circles under the eyes and headaches. Children with PANS often have fewer physiological and behavioral symptoms while on this diet.

Grounding

Being electrically grounded, also known as "earthing" or "grounding," naturally discharges and prevents chronic inflammation in the body by balancing the electrical potential between the body and the earth. This effect has massive health implications because of the well-established link between chronic inflammation and all chronic diseases and disorders, including PANS. The wearing of rubber-soled shoes prevents grounding; therefore, an easy way to ground is to walk barefoot on wet, outdoor, natural surfaces such as wet earth, wet grass or a beach shoreline.

Gut Dysbiosis

This imbalance in the gut microbiome *(see listing)* can lead to immune dysregulation *(see listing)*, nutritional deficiencies *(see listing)*, and cellular toxicities. "Dysbiosis" refers to a state of imbalance among the colonies of microorganisms (bacteria, yeast, viruses and parasites) within the gastrointestinal tract. Because 50-70% of the body's immune system is created by the gut microbiome, an imbalance can lead to a dysregulated immune system. Many children with PANS, as well as those with neurodevelopmental disorders *(see listing)*, allergies, asthma, autoimmune disorders and mood disorders have both gut dysbiosis and a dysregulated immune system. Many factors such as antibiotics *(see listing)*, a C-section birth, maternal inheritance, stress, the Standard American Diet *(see listing)*, GMO foods *(see listing)*, glyphosate *(see listing for Gluten)*, ibuprofen, Advil, Motrin and birth-control pills contribute to a dysbiotic microbiome.

Herbal Medicine

Medicinal herbs are plants with healing properties that are used to promote health and healing. Herbal medicine is the most ancient form of medicine known to humans, and many of today's pharmaceuticals were originally derived from herbs. Herbs are very different from drugs, however. While drugs suppress symptoms, herbs support and enhance the body's own natural healing processes. Herbal medicine uses substances extracted from flowers, fruits, roots, seeds and stems, either alone or together. Herbs commonly used for children with PANS include berberine, cat's claw (samento), stevia, olive leaf, oil of oregano, thyme and more. Children with PANS may benefit from the usage of herbal medicine as an alternative to pharmaceutical antibiotics *(see listing)*.

Herxheimer Reaction

Also known as "Jarisch–Herxheimer reaction," "Herxing" and "die off," this is a reaction to the release of toxins from the death of harmful microorganisms that happens when taking antibiotics *(see listing)* or anti-microbial remedies. Symptoms can include headache, nausea, fever, chills, low blood pressure, muscle pain and an increased heartbeat. Symptoms are usually not life-threatening and not prolonged.

Histamine

This neurotransmitter *(see listing)* is released by cells as part of an allergic response or as a response to injury. A histamine release typically causes rashes, itching, swelling and a stuffy nose. Most histamine in the body is produced in white blood cells called basophils and in mast cells *(see listing)*. A properly functioning liver *(see listing)* is necessary for the breakdown of histamine; therefore, a poorly functioning liver may lead to a longer occurrence of histamine-related symptoms. Healing the gut and improving liver function generally help with reducing histamine and inflammatory responses.

Holistic Medicine

Holistic medicine practitioners believe that the whole of the body is greater than the sum of its parts. Holistic practitioners consider all factors when treating illness, taking into account all of a patient's physical, mental, and social conditions in the treatment of illness. Children with PANS can benefit from working with a holistic practitioner.

Homeopathy

Homeopathy is a very gentle non-toxic way of treating the body, especially for the sensitive child. It is a type of energy medicine made from a diluted and succussed (shaken vigorously) tincture of a natural substance; substances used are flowers, plants, minerals, healthy tissue, animal venom, even diseases. After the tincture is created, it is poured over and absorbed by blank pellets or pills, dried, and placed in vials; these vials are known as homeopathic remedies. This diluted tincture contains an energetic imprint that resonates and supports the natural healing response, reversing or improving symptoms of illness. Through the dilution and succussion process, no actual substance remains inside the remedy; only the essence, the energy of the substance, remains. The gist of homeopathy is based on the theory that "like cures like." Children with PANS often benefit from homeopathic remedies such as constitutional remedies, nosode remedies *(see listing)* and series-therapy remedies.

Homotoxicology

This type of energy medicine is a way of detoxing the body utilizing homeopathy *(see listing)*, botanicals and nutritional supplements that detoxify and restore the body to normal health. Homotoxicology integrates the treatment principles of homeopathy with the diagnostic approach of allopathic medicine. It does not focus on the child's symptoms but rather on the underlying root causes which, in most cases, are the "homotoxins" that are disrupting the normal functioning of the body's biochemistry. The main principle of homotoxicology is to detoxify the body at a cellular level. Therefore, homotoxicology utilizes very complex homeopathic remedies to eliminate the toxins and restore the body to balance. Children with PANS often benefit from homotoxicology.

Hormone

This class of chemicals is produced in the body. Each hormone has a specific regulatory effect on the activity of certain cells or a certain organ or organs. *See also Neurotransmitter.*

Hypnotherapy

Hypnosis involves the induction of a trance-like state, in which the patient experiences an enhanced state of awareness. In this state, the conscious mind is suppressed, and the subconscious mind is more open to therapist suggestion. Through the use of guided imagery and repeated suggestion, hypnotherapy reduces negative thoughts and suppressed emotions so that behavioral change or symptom reduction can occur. Hypnosis is often used for conditions such as stress, anxiety and pain control.

Immune Dysregulation

A dysregulated (or dysfunctional) immune system is unable to protect a body from harmful environmental influences, and it can unleash a cascade of harmful effects upon the body. Examples of a dysregulated immune system include an over-reaction to an innocuous stimulus, an attack on the host's cells and tissues, an inability to detoxify, an inability to combat pathogenic (disease-causing) microbes, and an over-heightened state of attack. Any or all of these situations can lead to disruptions in cellular functions and operations. Children with PANS typically have immune dysregulation, which can be caused by gut dysbiosis *(see listing)*.

Immunoglobulin

These proteins in the serum and cells of the immune system function as antibodies *(see listing)*. They are produced by the immune system in response to the presence of toxins or foreign pathogens in the body called antigens. Antibodies contain specific binding sites that recognize and neutralize antigens. A type of therapy called Intravenous Immunoglobulin (IVIG; *see listing*) gives pooled immunoglobulin from donors as a treatment for people with weakened immune systems or other diseases. It is sometimes used as a Western medical treatment *(see listing)* for children with PANS.

Immunoglobulin A (IgA)

This type of antibody *(see listing)* plays a crucial role in the immune function of mucus membranes, which are found inside the gastrointestinal tract, nose, mouth, eyes, ears, lips, anus and vagina. Because these membranes are situated at openings to the body, IgA antibodies are the first line of defense against pathogens such as viruses and bacteria. High levels of IgA to specific foods *(see Food Sensitivity/Intolerance)* can be a sign that mucus membranes in the gut are damaged. Some children with PANS have been found to have an IgA deficiency.

Immunoglobulin E (IgE)

Although the body uses this type of antibody *(see listing)* to defend against certain parasites, IgE also plays a role in allergic asthma, food allergies and other allergic conditions. It is perhaps most well known in what are seen as "true," or anaphylactic, allergies to substances such as peanuts, tree nuts, insect bites, latex and other substances. IgE antibodies trigger the most powerful inflamma-tory reactions such as swelling of the throat or tongue, itchy rash, itchy throat, swelling of the eyes, vomiting, shortness of breath, low blood pressure and lightheadedness. An IgE reaction can be fatal, and people with a known IgE allergy will typically carry a form of injectable epinephrine with them at all times to counteract these fast-acting symptoms.

Immunoglobulin G (IgG)

This class of antibodies *(see listing)* is produced as part of natural exposure to food and is comprised of 70–75 different immuno-globulins. IgG-mediated reactions to food antigens are non-IgE (non-anaphylactic; *see listing for IgE*) allergies that can be classi-fied as a food sensitivity/intolerance *(see listing)*. IgG tests indi-cate a repeated exposure to food, which can be recognized by the body's immune system as a pathogen. Although the medical com-munity does not recommend clinical testing for IgG reactions as a diagnostic tool, anecdotal evidence from clinicians suggests that the removal and/or rotation of certain potential reaction-caus-ing foods such as gluten, dairy, corn, soy, peanuts, tree nuts, fish, shellfish, citrus and/or chocolate may be helpful in reducing some symptoms of children with PANS and other chronic conditions.

Immunoglobulin M (IgM)

This immunoglobulin is the first antibody *(see listing)* to respond during an infection. It is called the "natural antibody" because it can neutralize and clear new antigens without prior exposure. If IgM levels are low or negative and if IgG *(see listing)* levels are el-evated, then it is likely that the person had an infection sometime in the past to a specific antigen.

Integrative Medicine

This type of medicine is very similar to holistic medicine *(see listing)* in that it takes all aspects of lifestyle of a person (mind, body and spirit) into account. A variety of conventional and alternative heal-ing modalities or approaches are used, although these practitioners often prefer to use less-invasive interventions when possible.

Intestinal Permeability

Many children with PANS as well as those with neurodevelopmental disorders *(see listing)*, allergies, asthma, autoimmune conditions *(see listing)* and other chronic illnesses typically have what is known colloquially as a "leaky gut," or intestinal hyperpermeability. If a person has leaky gut, microscopic junctures between intestinal cells are too large to prevent fungal/bacterial derivatives, heavy metals and mal-digested food from reaching the blood and circulatory system. These toxins can greatly impair a child's behavior and development. Additionally, inefficient digestion of necessary nutrients can ravage neurological and immunological systems.

Intravenous Immunoglobulin (IVIG) Therapy

Intravenous Immunoglobulin therapy is a treatment for people with weakened immune systems or other diseases. IVIG pools antibodies *(see listing)* from different blood donors to provide antibodies that an individual is not making on their own. These pooled antibodies are delivered intravenously and are given to children and adults typically in spaced doses over a long period of time in order to fight off infections. It is sometimes used as a Western medical treatment *(see listing)* for children with PANS.

Jin Shin Jyutsu

This ancient art of harmonizing the flow of life energy ("chi") in the body was rediscovered in Japan in the early 1900's. The practice of it requires placing hands on one's own body or another's body. Jin shin jyutsu practitioners call this "jumper cabling" because one's "life battery" needs to be charged just like a car battery; hands are the "jumper cables" connecting the body to the universal energy flowing through everyone. Jin shin jyutsu is very nurturing, and people often experience a deep state of relaxation as built-up tension is released though gentle touch. Children with PANS can benefit from jin shin jyutsu because it can calm the nervous system, alleviate pain or discomfort from headaches, body tension or digestive issues, ease insomnia or anxiety *(see listing)*, improve attention and potentially strengthen the immune system.

K+ Channel Receptor Antibodies

A type of autoimmune encephalitis *(see listing)* known as Voltage-Gated Potassium Channel (VGKC) antibody-associated encephalitis is caused by the binding of antibodies *(see listing)* to voltage-gated potassium channel associated proteins, for which there is a blood test. This type of autoimmune encephalitis is typically treated with immunotherapy.

Leaky Gut Syndrome - *see Intestinal Permeability*

Learning Disability

This type of neurodevelopmental disorder *(see listing)* is marked by a severe difficulty in achieving grade-level academic performance. Dyslexia *(see listing)* is a reading disability, dyscalculia is a mathematics disability, and dysgraphia is a handwriting disability. A deterioration in handwriting ability is a potential symptom of PANS and usually shows up as more primitive handwriting, margin avoidance and/or margin drift. An auditory processing disorder is another type of learning disability that may appear in affected children. Children with neurodevelopmental disorders *(see listing)* such as autism *(see listing)*, ADD/ADHD *(see listing)* and Sensory Processing Disorder *(see listing)* often also have a learning disability. Learning disabilities can be improved by addressing root causes such as toxicity, gut dysbiosis *(see listing)*, immune dysregulation *(see listing)*, nutritional deficiencies *(see listing)*, hormonal imbalances and inflammation while implementing therapies that rewire the brain and central nervous system. Children with a learning disability often respond very well to vision therapy *(see listing for Vision)* and/or auditory therapy, if warranted.

Listening Therapy - *see Auditory Therapy*

Liver

The liver is the largest solid organ in the body, and it performs a variety of critical functions for the body such as the maintenance of blood-sugar levels; the detoxification of alcohol, drugs and environmental toxins; the manufacture of protein; the metabolization and storage of carbohydrates; the production and secretion of bile; the synthesis and secretion of certain hormones; the breakdown of histamine *(see listing)*; the synthesis, storage and processing of fats and cholesterol; and the filtering out of mutated hormones *(see listing)*. Children with PANS and other chronic health conditions often have sluggish livers. Symptoms of a sluggish liver can include constipation, abdominal bloating, skin rashes, blood-sugar fluctuations, mental fog, depression, and sensitivity to medications, fragrances and environmental toxins. *(See also Phase-One Detoxification, Phase-Two Detoxification and Phase-Three Detoxification.)*

Lyme Disease

Lyme disease is a tick-borne infectious disease known as *Borrelia burgdorferi* that is transmitted to humans by a black-legged deer tick; these ticks may carry up to twenty diseases. It was first reported in 1975 in the town of Old Lyme, Connecticut in the United States. There are five sub-species of *Borrelia burgdorferi*, and of these subspecies, there are more than 100 strains in the U.S. and 300 worldwide. In addition, there are common co-infections to Lyme disease; *Babesia, Bartonella, Ehrlichia, Mycoplasma* and herpetic viruses are the most common co-infections. Lyme disease is included in the umbrella term of PANS, and symptoms of chronic Lyme disease often mimic those of Rheumatoid Arthritis (RA). There is no definitive test for Lyme disease, although the IGeneX test and the Western Blot test *(see listing)* in combination with an ELISA test are often used; it is a clinical diagnosis.

Lysoganglioside GM1

A lysoganglioside is a lipid found in ganglion cells (nerve-cell clusters) in the brain as a component of cell plasma membranes. A test for autoantibodies directed against lysoganglioside GM1 is included in the Cunningham Panel *(see listing)*. These antibodies *(see listing)* may interfere with nervous-system function, especially motor-neuron function, and have been associated with neurologic conditions such as Guillain-Barre syndrome and PANS.

Malabsorption

This abnormality in the absorption of food and nutrients occurs in the gastrointestinal tract. It can develop from factors such as inflammation, stress, gastrointestinal infection, pH changes and/or a microbial imbalance known as gut dysbiosis *(see listing)*. When it is severe, malabsorption can lead to malnutrition, nutritional deficiencies *(see listing)* and a variety of anemias, such as iron-deficiency anemia and pernicious anemia. Children with PANS typically have malabsorption issues.

Mannose-Binding Lectin

This pattern-recognition protein of the innate immune system binds to a range of sugars, allowing it to interact with many different kinds of bacteria, viruses, yeasts, fungi and protozoa. It provides a first line of defense in the first hours/day of infection and may be especially important in a baby's immune-system development while the adaptive system is still immature. A deficiency of this protein is one of the most common human immunodeficiencies; an MBL deficiency increases the susceptibility of a person to infection. Some knowledgeable practitioners test for it as part of an evaluation of baseline immune system function for those with PANS.

Masgutova Method

This type of reflex integration occupational therapy is also called Neuro-Sensory-Motor and Reflex Integration (MNRI). It identifies retained primitive reflexes *(see listing)* in children then seeks to inhibit them through a series of prescribed movements. Children with developmental delays and neurodevelopmental disorders *(see listing)* typically have retained reflexes, but children with PANS can have them as well. They are caused by neurological damage from stress, trauma or toxic assault during a child's development and can cause a myriad of learning, behavioral, physical and mood problems. Children with retained reflexes may have problems with coordination, balance, concentration, impulse control, sensory perceptions, fine motor skills, gross motor skills, sleep, immunity, energy levels, social learning, emotional learning and academic learning.

Mast-Cell Activation

Mast cells are a type of white-blood cell known as mastocytes (leukocytes). They become activated due to an allergic reaction, an immune reaction or a response to triggers such as emotional stress, or other kinds of stress such as temperature changes, pollution, pollen, dander, fatigue, odors, venom, infections, sunlight, certain foods, alcohol and medications. Mast cells do not just release histamine *(see listing)*; instead, they release their contents into surrounding tissues. Mast-cell activation can look like a histamine intolerance, but with a mast-cell activation there are many more triggers for activation than happens with a histamine intolerance. Symptoms of mast-cell activation can include symptoms of anaphylaxis such as swelling of the throat or tongue, itchy rash, itchy throat, swelling of the eyes, vomiting, shortness of breath, low blood pressure and lightheadedness *(see Immunoglobulin E)*. In addition, blood-brain-barrier permeability can occur from activation of these cells. A child with allergies, eczema, asthma, an autoimmune disease *(see listing)* or other type of chronic inflammation may be vulnerable to an onset of PANS because of mast-cell activation. Children with mast-cell activation or histamine intolerance can benefit from a low-histamine diet.

Melatonin

Melatonin is a hormone *(see listing)* that is produced in every cell in the body, but the major source comes from the pineal gland. When melatonin is released from the pineal gland, it aids in synchronizing the body's internal circadian clock and daily rhythm in different parts of the body, with peak levels occurring at nighttime. Melatonin regulates the sleep/wake cycle by making the person drowsy and lowering the body temperature. Melatonin's response to light and darkness is very important for sleep cycles; the production of it is suppressed when exposed to blue light, which is found both in daylight and light from video devices. Therefore, it is important to eliminate exposure to video devices after the sun goes down. In addition, when stress (especially chronic stress) and anxiety *(see listing)* increase, cortisol levels will rise, the adrenal glands can become fatigued and the hypothalamic-pituitary-adrenal axis becomes dysfunctional. This domino effect decreases the body's production of melatonin and alters the body's natural circadian rhythms. Many children with PANS have poor sleep patterns.

Meridian

Life-force energy, known as "chi," travels along these pathways in the body. Although Western medical practitioners typically do not recognize these pathways as they cannot be confirmed with scientific evidence, the concept of them has been around for thousands of years in Traditional Chinese Medicine. Acupuncture *(see listing)*, acupressure *(see listing)*, and other types of energy medicine and therapies also use the concept of meridians.

Microbiome

The collection of genomes of microbes living in the gastrointestinal tract is known as the microbiome; microbiota are the organisms (bacteria, yeasts, parasites and viruses) living within the microbiome. The entire digestive tract is a living ecological community of microorganisms of over 100 trillion bacteria. Roughly 50-70% of the body's immune system is created by the gut's microbiota. Children with PANS typically have an impaired microbiome, known as gut dysbiosis *(see listing)*, and this typically leads to immune dysregulation *(see listing)*.

Minerals

Many of these building blocks of rocks are essential for human health as they aid in detoxification, serve as building blocks for bones and teeth, help regulate the immune system, feed the adrenal glands, thyroid and other glands, and serve as catalysts for metabolic processes. Children with PANS are often deficient in minerals such as magnesium, zinc and iodine as well as trace minerals due to a combination of picky or restrictive eating, the Standard American Diet *(see listing)*, gut dysbiosis *(see listing)*, stress and other factors.

Mitochondrial Dysfunction

Mitochondrial dysfunction occurs when the mitochondria, the "powerhouses of the cells," are not able to do their job due to genetic or environmental factors. The following symptoms are common in children with mitochondrial dysfunction: large motor delays, failure to thrive, growth delays, low muscle tone, extreme fatigue, an inability to regulate temperature, autistic symptoms *(see listing)*, global muscle weakness and difficulty waking. However, some researchers now believe that all chronic conditions, including PANS, have some level of mitochondrial dysfunction.

Molecular Mimicry

A structural, functional or immunological similarity between certain pathogens and specific human proteins may lead to immune cross-reactivity due to molecular mimicry, in which the immune system mistakes these proteins for the pathogens, essentially causing autoimmune disease *(see listing)*.

Motor Cortex

This part of the brain is located in the cerebral cortex and is responsible for the planning, control, and execution of voluntary movements.

MTHFR Genetic Mutation/SNP

MTHFR (MethyleneTetraHydroFolate Reductase) is an enzyme encoded by the MTHFR gene, which is responsible for making folate (vitamin B_9). Folate can cross the blood-brain barrier whereas the synthetic form, folic acid, cannot. Folate is needed to make the brain methylate; put simply, methylation is a method of detoxification. Children with PANS, neurodevelopmental disorders *(see listing)* and other chronic health conditions are more apt to have a defect of this gene; medical researchers have discovered that exposure to environmental toxins are associated with the defect. A defect in the methylation process can affect speech, language, auditory processing, reading comprehension, focus, concentration, socialization, DNA repair, homocysteine levels, inflammation and the recycling of key antioxidants such as glutathione *(see listing)*. Under a health practitioner's guidance, children with this defect often take methylated forms of supplements such as methycobalamin, pyridoxal phosphate, dimethylglycine, folinic acid/folate and trimethylglycine to improve their ability to methylate.

Muscle Testing - *see Applied Kinesiology*

Mycotoxin

These toxic secondary metabolites are a subset of biotoxins that are produced by fungi, including molds and yeasts. Mycotoxins damage the immune system and can cause symptoms such as sneezing, headaches, fatigue, nosebleeds, body aches, shortness of breath, memory loss, sinus congestion, sore throat, coughing, confusion, brain fog, vision impairment, dizziness, anxiety *(see listing)*, sleep problems and seizures. Exposure to mold and mycotoxins can cause some of the same symptom as PANS, especially those of Lyme disease and its coinfections. Because of a dysregulated immune system *(see listing for Immune Dysregulation)*, exposure to mycotoxins can leave a child more susceptible to PANS, and having PANS can leave a child more susceptible to harm from mycotoxins. Mycotoxins can activate a state in which TH17 cells *(see listing)* proliferate, which is helpful during acute infection; however, uncontrolled TH17 activity is associated with autoimmune pathology. Mycotoxin exposure can be determined with a urine test. In addition, the visual contrast sensitivity test is a useful online screening tool to check for mycotoxin exposure, and Mycometrics' Environmental Relative Moldiness Index (ERMI) is a well-regarded tool for evaluating the presence of mold inside a building. In addition, Ritchie Shoemaker MD has developed testing to look for genetic susceptibility to mycotoxins, such as the markers C3a, C4a, MMP-9, MSH, TGF-β1, VEGP and VIP. Some physicians use off-label cholestyramine to bind and remove biotoxins from the body, while other practitioners use other therapies and approaches.

Myofunctional Therapy

This program of specific exercises targeting facial muscles used to chew and swallow can strengthen the tongue. Children with PANS, especially those with tongue tie, may benefit from working with a team including a myofunctional therapist, a functional dentist and an osteopathic physician *(see listing for Osteopathy)*. This team can address oro-facial structural abnormalities that prevent muscles, bones, and teeth in the cranial complex from reaching their more complete genetic potential. Oro-facial abnormalities can cause restricted breathing, sleep apnea, poor concentration, hyperactivity, speech delays, sleep disturbances, headaches, feeding issues and irritability.

N-AcetylCysteine (NAC)

N-Acetyl Cysteine is an altered version of the amino acid cysteine. NAC is an antioxidant that helps boost production of glutathione *(see listing)*, an antioxidant that removes oxygen radicals from cells. Glutathione is an important antioxidant produced by the body that helps reduce free radical damage and plays a role in the detoxification of harmful substances and heavy metals. Children with PANS may benefit from the supplementation of NAC under the guidance of their healthcare practitioner.

Naturopathy (Naturopathic Medicine)

This type of holistic medicine uses the healing power of nature. Naturopathic doctors (NDs) are typically trained to look at the root causes of chronic health conditions such as toxicity, lymphatic drainage problems, gut dysbiosis *(see listing)*, immune dysregulation *(see listing)*, nutritional deficiencies *(see listing)*, hormonal imbalances and inflammation as well as how the mind and spirit affect the body. Naturopaths use a variety of non-pharmaceutical interventions such as herbal medicine *(see listing)*, homeopathy *(see listing)*, and dietary and lifestyle change recommendations as well as nutritional supplementation to help a client achieve a state of more optimal health.

Neurodevelopmental Disorder

This class of disorders includes autism *(see listing)*, ADD/ADHD *(see listing)*, Sensory Processing Disorder *(see listing)* and learning disabilities *(see listing)*, including dyslexia *(see listing)*. These are whole-body disorders that affect both the brain and the body; they should no longer be thought of as mental disorders. There are no definitive blood tests for these disorders; instead, practitioners such as neurologists typically make a diagnosis after observation of a child's symptoms. Western medicine is beginning to understand that neurodevelopmental disorders may be related to anomalies in the gut microbiome *(see listing)*, immune dysregulation *(see listing)*, nutritional deficiencies *(see listing)*, vision processing *(see listing for Vision)*, auditory processing, sensory processing *(see listing)*, retained primitive reflexes *(see listing)*, neurotransmitter imbalances *(see listing)*, food sensitivities/intolerances *(see listing)*, and environmental toxins. More knowledgeable practitioners now believe that a large percentage of children with neurodevelopmental disorders may also have PANS. Children can lose their diagnosis by addressing the root causes of toxicity, gut dysbiosis *(see listing)*, immune dysregulation *(see listing)*, nutritional deficiencies, hormonal imbalances and inflammation while implementing therapies that rewire the brain and central nervous system.

Neurofeedback

This non-invasive, computer-aided technique trains the brain to regulate itself by giving feedback, both visual and auditory. If the client's brain produces brain-wave patterns (measured by sensors applied to the head) that a practitioner has determined will help the client, then they receive reinforcement. If the client does not produce those patterns, then they do not receive visual and auditory reinforcement. The subconscious brain wants reinforcement and therefore will automatically adjust brain-wave function. By adjusting brain-wave patterns in this way over a period of time through these sessions, clients may experience a reduction of symptoms, including improved concentration, focus, stamina, organizational skills, time-management skills and academic skills as well as less depression, anxiety *(see listing)*, tics *(see listing)*, anger, obsessiveness *(see listing for OCD)* and behavioral problems. Research supports that these changes are lasting. There are over 3,000 peer-reviewed studies to support the efficacy of neurofeedback for a variety of conditions. Children with PANS often benefit from using neurofeedback.

Neurotransmitters

These chemical messengers transmit nerve impulses. Two types are important for children with PANS: Amino acids and monoamines. Glutamate, GABA, aspartate, glycine and D-serine are amino-acid transmitters, while dopamine, norepinephrine, epinephrine, serotonin and histamine are monoamines. *(See separate entry listings for Glutamate, GABA, Dopamine, Serotonin and Histamine).* Children with PANS often have neurotransmitter imbalances of these two types. Neurotransmitter imbalances often begin in the gastrointestinal tract, both because intestinal microbes play a critical role in the production and metabolism of neurotransmitters and also because nutritional precursors to neurotransmitters are derived from the gut. Healing gut dysbiosis *(see listing)*, changing the composition of the diet away from the Standard American Diet *(see listing)* and supplementing with targeted neurotransmitters under a health practitioner's guidance can often alleviate some symptoms of mood or behavioral problems associated with PANS.

NMDA Receptor

The N-methyl-D-aspartate receptor (also known as the NMDA receptor) is a glutamate *(see listing)* receptor found in nerve cells. It is activated when the amino acids glutamate and glycine bind to it. NMDA receptors have been implicated by a number of studies to be strongly involved with excitotoxicity *(see listing)*, the process by which nerve cells are damaged or killed by excessive stimulation by neurotransmitters such as glutamate. Excitotoxicity can cause encephalopathy and seizures. A blood test can confirm the diagnosis of NMDAR antibody encephalitis *(see listing for Anti-NMDA Receptor Encephalitis).*

Nosode Remedy

This type of homeopathic remedy *(see listing)* is made from pathogens such as *Mycoplasma*, Epstein-Barr virus, *Streptococcus, Bartonella, Borrelia* and *Babesia* to combat stubborn infections resulting from the pathogens. They can be very helpful to a child with PANS, especially when given in series-therapy form.

Nutrient

Vitamins, minerals and other substances are common form of nutrients, and they are needed to keep the body healthy, grow, repair tissue, produce energy, detoxify and perform other bodily functions. Nutrients are essential, meaning that they cannot be produced within the body and must be consumed in the form of food or supplements.

Nutritional Deficiency

These insufficiencies of essential vitamins, minerals and other nutrients are common in children with PANS. Common causes of nutritional deficiencies are gut dysbiosis *(see listing)*, inflammation, picky eating, maternal inheritance and toxicity. If nutritional deficiencies occur during childhood, they can contribute to neuro-developmental disorders *(see listing)*, developmental delays, failure to thrive, growth delays and chronic health conditions.

Obsessive Compulsive Disorder (OCD)

This type of anxiety disorder is a common symptom of PANS. It is characterized by unreasonable thoughts and fears (obsessions) that lead a child to perform repetitive behaviors (compulsions) to help relieve or manage anxious, fearful, or worrying feelings. A child often consciously knows these thoughts and behaviors are unreasonable, which can increase levels of stress and anxiety *(see listing)*. In order to be diagnosed with OCD, these obsessions and compulsions have to be uncontrollable and an individual has to spend a significant amount of time everyday in mental or physical rituals.

Occipital Lobe

This part of the cerebral cortex of the brain is responsible for processing visual information from the eyes, otherwise known as vision processing. *(See listing for Vision).*

Occludin

This protein, along with other molecules, is required for the formation of the blood-brain barrier *(see listing)*. Viruses or bacteria can induce degradation of occludin, and testing for antibodies to it is a marker of blood-brain-barrier dysfunction.

Oppositional Defiant Disorder (ODD)

This type of behavior disorder in children and teenagers is defined as a pattern of defiant, hostile, argumentative or noncompliant behaviors toward adults or authority figures. Children with this disorder typically have angry and irritable moods, as well as argumentativeness, vindictive behaviors and noncompliant behaviors that are much more frequent, extreme and disruptive than normal. These children and teens are easily irritated and lack introspection about their behaviors. Children with ODD may have an undiagnosed case of PANS.

Oral Allergy Syndrome

Also known as Pollen-Food Allergy, Oral Allergy Syndrome is an allergic reaction in the mouth when eating food, usually uncooked fruits or vegetables. It is typically only seen in people with seasonal allergies to tree pollen.

Osteopathy (Osteopathic Medicine)

This form of healthcare stresses the relationship between the body's form and function as well as its ability to heal by looking at the whole person. Doctors of Osteopathy (DO) are fully qualified physicians that are licensed to prescribe medication as well as perform surgery in all 50 states of the United States. In addition to doing internships and residency training in standard allopathic medicine *(see listing)*, they also receive special training in the musculoskeletal system and in the manual and physical manipulation of the body.

Oxidative Stress

This condition occurs when there is an imbalance between free radicals and antioxidants in the body. It can be caused by a variety of things such as exposure to toxins, exposure to pathogens, emotional stress and antioxidant deficiencies, which are common in the Standard American Diet *(see listing)*. Common antioxidants used for rectifying this imbalance are glutathione *(see listing)*, omega-3 fatty acids, curcumin, vitamin C and N-AcetylCysteine *(see listing)*.

Parasympathetic Nervous System

This part of the autonomic nervous system is responsible for the state of "feed and breed" (also known as "rest and digest") within the body; it is the calming aspect of the nervous system. Children with PANS, as well as those with neurodevelopmental disorders *(see listing)*, mood disorders and behavior disorders often have cranial-nerve damage stemming from trauma, stress, toxic assault, brain infection or brain inflammation that prevent them from being in a parasympathetic-dominant state. Children with these conditions can benefit from calming activities such as yoga, meditation, extending exhales longer than inhales, tai chi *(see listing)*, jin shin jyutsu *(see listing)* and qi gong *(see listing)*. They can also benefit from therapies such as biofeedback *(see listing)*, neurofeedback *(see listing)*, PEMF *(see listing)*, EMDR *(see listing)*, craniosacral therapy *(see listing)*, Masgutova Method reflex integration *(see listing)*, Anat Baniel therapy *(see listing)* and Blomberg Rhythmic Movement Training *(see listing)*. In addition, a low-glutamate diet *(see listing for Glutamate)*, a non-Standard American Diet *(see listing)*, avoidance of food allergies/sensitivities *(see listing)*, supplementation with GABA *(see listing)* and other targeted supplements, and addressing the infectious and toxic agents contributing to PANS can help a child be more parasympathetic dominant, thus allowing the body to better heal.

Parietal Lobe

This part of the cerebral cortex of the brain is responsible for processing sensory information having to do with taste, temperature, and touch.

Pediatric Acute-onset Neuropsychiatric Syndrome (PANS)

In PANS, an infectious trigger such as Lyme, *Streptococcus*, or *Bartonella*, environmental factors or other possible triggers cross the blood-brain barrier *(see listing)* and create an autoimmune and inflammatory response that impacts the brain. These infections typically occur in childhood. PANS is often suspected if a child quickly begins to exhibit life-changing symptoms such as OCD *(see listing)*, severe restrictive eating, anxiety *(see listing)*, tics *(see listing)*, personality changes, decline in math and handwriting abilities, and sensitivities to sensory input *(see listing for Sensory Processing Disorder)*. These behaviors and psychiatric issues can come on with such intensity that they are often completely debilitating.

Pediatric Autoimmune Neuropsychiatric Disorder Associated with Streptococcal Infection (PANDAS)

This term is used to describe children who have a rapid onset of anxiety *(see listing)*, psychosis *(see listing)*, sleep disturbances, depression *(see listing)*, anorexia *(see listing)*, Obsessive Compulsive Disorder *(see listing)*, Oppositional Defiant Disorder *(see listing)*, and/or tics *(see listing)*. The condition is thought to be due to an autoimmune response to a *Strep* infection that crosses the blood-brain barrier *(see listing)*, resulting in a dysregulated immune response *(see listing for Immune Dysregulation)*. The body produces antibodies to the *Strep* bacteria, affecting the basal ganglia *(see listing)* in the brain, which control the body's movement and behavior, thus creating some of the symptoms commonly seen in this condition.

Pediatric Infection-Triggered Autoimmune Neuropsychiatric Disorders (PITAND)

This disorder is characterized by the development of OCD *(see listing)*, tics *(see listing)*, and neuropsychiatric symptoms after a viral or bacterial infection. PITAND is similar to PANDAS except that it can be caused by any pathogen; they are both subsets of PANS.

Phase-One Detoxification

This process of clearing toxins from the liver *(see listing)* includes the oxidation, reduction and hydrolysis of functional groups on drug, chemical and other toxic molecules. In layman's terms, this is akin to putting garbage into garbage bags. When there are too many substances to detoxify, the liver becomes overwhelmed.

Phase-Two Detoxification

This process of clearing toxins from the liver *(see listing)* is known as the conjugation pathway because the liver adds substances like the aminoacid glycine to toxins processed in phase one to make them harmless, which makes it easy for the body to excrete and remove them. In layman's terms, this is akin to a garbage man carrying away garbage bags full of garbage.

Phase-Three Detoxification

Researchers have recently discovered another detoxification process that is mostly in the small intestine. This process, known as antiporter activity, happens both before phase-one detoxification *(see listing)* and after phase-two detoxification *(see listing)*. Gut dysbiosis *(see listing)* and inflammation may interfere with these processes; thus, a gut-healing diet and probiotic supplementation may improve normal detoxification processes.

Phospholipid

This type of fat contains a phosphate group; lecithin, phosphatidylcholine and phosphatidylserine *(see listing)* are examples of phospholipids. Phospholipids form the basic structure of cell membranes and are critical to a cell's ability to function. Children with PANS as well as those with neurodevelopmental disorders *(see listing)* and mitochondrial dysfunction *(see listing)* are often given phospholipids to repair their cell membranes and improve symptoms of mitochondrial dysfunction such as fatigue, low muscle tone and impaired cognitive abilities.

Phosphatidylserine

This type of phospholipid *(see listing)* is a component of cell membranes. It plays an important part in mental functions such as focus, attention and memory, and it can help with impulse control and hyperactivity. Healthcare practitioners sometimes recommend it to children with neurodevelopmental disorders *(see listing)* and PANS and also to adults with Alzheimer's.

Plasma

This yellow-colored liquid is a component of blood that holds blood cells in suspension; it is the extracellular matrix of blood cells. Because blood plasma contains antibodies *(see listing)*, it is removed and replaced during the rare procedure of plasmapheresis *(see listing)* to improve symptoms of PANS, autism *(see listing)* and other autoimmune disorders *(see listing)*.

Plasmapheresis

This is a process by which blood containing harmful autoantibodies is removed from the body and then replaced with "clean blood." The procedure involves taking whole blood from a person, separating it into plasma *(see listing)* and blood cells, removing the plasma, and replacing it with another solution, such as saline, albumin, or donor plasma. The new solution is then returned to the patient. It is sometimes Western medicine's therapy of last resort for patients with PANS, autism *(see listing)* and other autoimmune disorders *(see listing)*. While symptoms can improve quickly for some recipients of this procedure, it may have a less impactful effect on others and is generally reserved for the most severe cases due to the invasive and costly nature of the procedure. Caution is warranted in the use of donor plasma, as not all toxins or infectious agents are removed before being given to a recipient.

Post-Traumatic Stress Disorder (PTSD)

This is a disorder in which a person has difficulty recovering after experiencing or witnessing some kind of personally terrifying event. The trauma can be from war trauma, natural disaster experience, or abuse, but it can also result from events such as medical experiences and grief. PTSD symptoms can last for weeks, years, or even a lifetime if not addressed and can affect how the brain and body function. Symptoms may include nightmares, unwanted memories, avoidance of situations that bring back memories, heightened reactions, poor attention, poor cognitive functioning, behavioral issues, sensory-processing problems, physical pain, anxiety *(see listing)* and mood-regulation issues. People with PTSD are often in a state of sympathetic-nervous-system dominance ("fight or flight;" *see listing for Sympathetic Nervous System*) or even a dorsal-vagal state of withdrawal.

Primitive Reflexes

These neurodevelopmental reflexes develop as a way to help a baby grow and mature in utero and during the first year of life. Examples of primitive reflexes are those for breastfeeding, grasping, crawling and flight or fight. As babies mature, they develop postural reflexes that are much more mature patterns of reflexes to help control balance, coordination and sensorimotor development. In some cases, babies retain their primitive reflexes, known as retained reflexes, past the first year of life because they fail to integrate them well with the rest of their nervous system. These delays can cause developmental delays and can result from adverse reactions to toxins, birth trauma, C-section birth and other factors. Retained reflexes are exceedingly common in children with ADD/ADHD *(see listing)*, autism *(see listing)*, Sensory Processing Disorder *(see listing)* and learning disabilities *(see listing)*. Children with PANS may also have retained primitive reflexes. Specialized occupational therapists such as those trained in the Masgutova Method *(see listing)*, Blomberg Rhythmic Movement *(see listing)* or Brain Balance can determine which reflexes are retained and help to integrate them.

Probiotic

This type of supplement contains live bacteria and/or yeasts that can improve intestinal health as well as overall health by restoring balance in the microbiome. Children with PANS often have gut dysbiosis *(see listing)*, and supplementing with probiotics can re-establish colonies of beneficial bacteria and yeasts that produce certain vitamins, detoxify the body, defend against pathogenic invaders and perform other important functions that are critical for optimal health.

Procedural Learning

This type of learning is created by repeating a complex activity over and over again. It creates a "groove" in the brain's neural network so that a person does not have to think consciously about doing the activity. Examples of activities learned with procedural learning are riding a bike and tying shoes.

Psychiatrist

This type of medical doctor (MD) specializes in the diagnosis and treatment of mental disorders and receives training beyond typical medical training in order to specialize in psychiatry. These practitioners may use a variety of therapies but often prescribe medication to manage symptoms of mental health disorders.

Psychologist

This type of clinician holds a graduate degree with advanced training in behavioral problems, emotional disturbances, and the diagnosis and treatment of diseases of the brain; in most states, they cannot prescribe medication. They often work in clinical practice but may also do research, teach, or provide developmental or educational assessments. In a clinical setting, a psychologist may use Cognitive Behavioral Therapy *(see listing)*, "talk therapy," or other non-invasive modalities to treat clients. These practitioners will often refer to a psychiatrist or other medical doctor if they believe that medication is necessary.

Psychosis

In this mental state, a person is experiencing some loss of contact with reality. When this occurs, it is called a psychotic episode. With psychosis, a person's thoughts and perceptions are disturbed, and the individual may have difficulty understanding what is real and what is not. Symptoms of psychosis include delusions and hallucinations, which can cause agitated behaviors. A person experiencing psychosis may also display incoherent speech and odd behavior, as well as depression *(see listing)*, anxiety *(see listing)*, sleep problems, withdrawn behaviors, and generalized difficulty functioning. Some children with PANS may experience psychosis.

Psychotherapist

These clinicians hold a graduate degree and a state license to engage clients in "talk therapy" or other non-invasive, therapeutic modalities to improve a client's quality of life; they cannot prescribe medication. Clients often can achieve greater functioning in society, greater satisfaction in relationships, improved performance in work or play, and greater general psychological health and well-being. Psychotherapists are typically Licensed Professional Counselors (LPC), Licensed Marriage and Family Therapists (LMFT), or Licensed Clinical Social Workers (LCSW).

Pulsed Electromagnetic Field Therapy (PEMF)

Pulsed Electromagnetic Field therapy (PEMF) is a way to alter bio-electromagnetic fields to enhance cellular functioning and communication, which in turn can enhance self-healing and wellness. Controlled and pulsed electromagnetic frequencies can deliver health-enhancing EMFs to the cells to stimulate electrical and chemical processes in bodily tissues. PEMF is used to support those with conditions such as anxiety *(see listing)*, injury, chronic pain, infectious disease and autoimmune disease *(see listing)*. Children with PANS may benefit from the use of PEMF therapy.

Qi Gong

Qi gong exercises can balance and harness qi ("chi") or "life energy." This type of practice is frequently described as "meditation in motion" because it entails meditation, breathing, slow movement and breathing. Qi gong can be helpful for children with PANS as well as those with neurodevelopmental disorders *(see listing)*, pain, anxiety *(see listing)*, OCD *(see listing)*, balance disorders, sleep issues, mood disorders and autoimmune disorders *(see listing)*.

Quantum Electroencephalography (QEEG) / Brain Map

Electroencephalography (EEG) is the measurement of electrical patterns at the surface of the scalp that reflect cortical activity; these are commonly referred to as "brainwaves." A QEEG is an EEG brain map that is a non-invasive and painless process. A cap with sensors that record the brain's electrical activity is placed on the head, and data is recorded with the individual's eyes open as well as closed. This data is compared against a reference database of other people's data. The analysis identifies and highlights variations from the norm and gives information about issues impacting brain functioning through pattern analysis. Distinct EEG patterns are used to identify anomalies such as attention deficits *(see listing)*, depression *(see listing)*, inflammation and anxiety *(see listing)*.

Quantum Reflex Analysis (QRA)

This type of analysis is a form of O-ring kinesiology *(see listing)* testing developed by Dr. Bob Marshall. QRA differentiates itself from other techniques because of its reliance on palpating targeted acupressure *(see listing)* points as a means of assessing the relative strength or weakness of an organ in relation to stressors or balancers in the field.

S100-B

These calcium-binding proteins play an important role in normal development and recovery after injury of the central nervous system, including the brain. They are a useful biomarker of brain damage because they measure glial activation and/or death in many disorders of the central nervous system, including PANS. A test for antibodies to S100-B can test for blood-brain-barrier *(see listing)* dysfunction.

Sensory Processing Disorder (SPD)

Children with Sensory Processing Disorder have great difficulty processing and acting upon information received through their senses. There are eight senses involved in a child's development that are necessary for processing information: Hearing, touch, taste, smell, vision, vestibular, proprioception (muscle and joint movement and sense of self) and interoception (the understanding by the self to feel what is going on inside the body). Children with SPD may be over- or under-sensitive to lights, sounds and textures, may lack the ability to orient themselves properly in space, and may have difficulty controlling their movements. SPD can be a standalone neurodevelopmental disorder *(see listing)*, but it is also commonly seen in children with autism *(see listing)*, ADD/ADHD *(see listing)*, learning disabilities *(see listing)* and PANS. Children can lose their diagnosis of Sensory Processing Disorder by addressing the root causes of toxicity, gut dysbiosis *(see listing)*, immune dysregulation *(see listing)*, nutritional deficiencies *(see listing)*, hormonal imbalances and inflammation while implementing therapies that rewire the brain and central nervous system.

Serotonin

This neurotransmitter *(see listing)* is derived from the amino acid tryptophan and aids in the control of appetite, sleep cycles and mood. A serotonin deficiency is linked to depression *(see listing)*, impaired attention span and social withdrawal. Because it is made in the gastrointestinal tract, a person with gut dysbiosis *(see listing)* may have lower levels of serotonin.

Severe Combined ImmunoDeficiency (SCID)

This rare genetic disorder is characterized by the disturbed development of functional T cells *(see listing)* and B cells *(see listing)*, resulting in defective antibody response. It is also known as Glanzmann–Riniker syndrome, alymphocytosis, thymic alymphoplasia and severe mixed immunodeficiency syndrome.

Short-Chain Fatty Acid

All fatty acids are both important structural components for cells as well as important dietary sources of fuel; they are not the same thing as fat. Short-chain fatty acids are produced when dietary fiber is fermented in the colon. Butyric acid is an example of a short-chain fatty acid; it is reparative in the gut, can cross the blood-brain barrier and can get inside cells. A lack of good fats entering the diet, as is common in the Standard American Diet *(see listing)*, means that there are not enough good fats entering cells to push out toxins. Children with PANS often have a short-chain-fatty-acid deficiency.

Somatic Symptom

This type of symptom is experienced in the body as a physical sensation; "soma" is the Greek word for body. Children with PANS often experience somatic symptoms such as headaches, nausea, dizziness, pain and fatigue.

Sound Stimulation

This type of auditory therapy, also known as Auditory Training, is based on the work of the French ear, nose and throat specialist, Dr. Alfred Tomatis. Sound Stimulation delivers electronically modified music through specialized equipment to improve auditory-processing issues. Children with PANS and neurodevelopmental disorders *(see listing)* often have auditory-processing difficulties and may benefit from this type of therapy.

SPECT Scan

A Single Photon Emission Computed Tomography (SPECT) scan is a type of nuclear imaging test that produces 3-D images that show how blood flows to the arteries and veins in the brain; it combines computed tomography (CT) with a radioactive tracer. It is sometimes used by physicians for children with neurodevelopmental disorders *(see listing)* and adults with Alzheimer's to discover underperforming parts of the brain, which are receiving less blood flow.

Standard American Diet

This type of diet typically is high in processed foods and low in nutrients. Processed foods can contain unhealthy vegetable oils, trans fats, artificial colors, artificial flavors, natural flavors, flavor enhancers and preservatives and flours that are refined to contain very little fiber or complex carbohydrates. Each of these types of ingredients has been shown to decrease health. Processed foods are also typically low in vegetables and high in GMO ingredients *(see listing)*, pesticides and ingredients that many children with PANS may have food sensitivities/intolerances *(see listing)* to such as gluten *(see listing)*, dairy, corn, soy and eggs.

Strabismus

Strabismus, commonly known as crossed or wall eyes, is a visual condition that affects the ability of the eyes and the brain to communicate. One eye correctly aims at an object while the other eye aims above, below or to the side of it, causing double vision. The brain struggles to integrate competing messages, causing disorganization and confusion within the brain. Children with PANS and neurodevelopmental disorders *(see listing)* can sometimes have strabismus, and this condition can often be corrected without surgery through the implementation of vision therapy *(see listing for Vision)* by a developmental optometrist *(see listing)*.

Strep Titer

These antibody *(see listing)* blood-titer tests can show immunological evidence of a past *Strep* infection. The Anti-Streptolysin O (ASO) titer *(see listing)* typically rises three to six weeks after a *Strep* infection, while the DNaseB titer *(see listing)* rises six to eight weeks after an infection.

Supplements

These concentrated sources of vitamins *(see listing)*, minerals *(see listing)* and other nutrients *(see listing)* and substances can enhance a person's daily diet. Because many children with PANS have gut dysbiosis *(see listing)* and are picky eaters, they may not be getting enough daily nutrients and may need to consume supplements in order to improve health status by addressing nutritional deficiencies *(see listing)* and/or maintaining a proper balance of certain nutrients. Although supplements come in many forms such as liquids, capsules, gel capsules and hard tablets, knowledgeable practitioners are more apt not to recommend hard tablets, as their form does not dissolve as well as the other forms inside the body.

Sydenham Chorea

This neurological disorder typically occurs in children aged five to 15 years of age, and it results from infection via Group A Beta-Hemolytic *Streptococcus* (GABHS), the bacterium that causes rheumatic fever. Symptoms of the disorder include muscular weakness, uncoordinated movements, slurred speech, stumbling, falling, emotional instability and a difficulty in concentrating and writing. Symptoms are caused by the reaction to the bacterium as it affects the basal ganglia *(see listing)*, which control movement.

Sympathetic Nervous System

This part of the autonomic nervous system is responsible for the state of "fight or flight." This state causes a rush of adrenaline (epinephrine) to the muscles, an increase in heart rate and a shutdown of digestive processes. In the modern world with its high level of stress, many people are in a chronic state of sympathetic dominance. In addition, children with PANS, neurodevelopmental disorders *(see listing)*, mood disorders, autoimmune disorders *(see listing)* and other chronic conditions are often in this chronic state. Some of this is due to stress from external factors such as emotional stress and being pressured for time, while some of it is due to cranial-nerve damage from internalized toxins. Other contributory factors include exposure to EMFs *(see listing)*, consumption of the Standard American Diet *(see listing)*, poor sleep habits *(see listing for Melatonin)*, sensory-processing difficulties *(see listing for Sensory Processing Disorder)* and infections such as PANS. Many of these children have a retained Moro primitive reflex *(see listing for Primitive Reflexes)* that can cause free-floating anxiety *(see listing)*. A person in a chronic state of sympathetic dominance may likely have adrenal fatigue, which can affect the body's ability to regulate sleep, inflammation, blood sugar and hormone *(see listing)* production. See the listing for *Parasympathetic Nervous System* for suggestions on returning to a parasympathetic "rest and digest" state.

Tai Chi

This ancient mind-body healing practice was developed in China centuries ago. Although it is a martial art, it is typically practiced for its health benefits such as reduction of anxiety *(see listing)* and improved balance. The slow-flowing movement is practiced to move the body's "chi" (energy) in a healthful way. Children with PANS may benefit from the practice of tai chi.

Tapping – *see EFT/Tapping*

T Cells

T lymphocytes, known as "T cells," are a type of lymphocyte (small, white blood cells) that does some of the work of the immune system. They mature in the thymus and are the equivalent of the firefighters who organize and put the fire out. In immune disorders such as PANS, there is an over-proliferation of B cells *(see listing)* and not enough T cells that can organize and stop the cause of the immune-system attack.

Temporal Lobe

This part of the cerebral cortex of the brain is responsible for processing auditory information. Its function is to understand sound in a meaningful way. Damage to this lobe can affect short-term memory and the ability to stay on task.

Thalamus

This part of the forebrain lies below the corpus callosum, and it is essentially the director of sensory information within the brain. It receives sensory information from parts of the body such as the ears, eyes and skin and then relays these signals to areas of the brain where it can be processed. The thalamus is linked to the basal ganglia *(see listing)*, which facilitate movement and inhibit competing movements. A disruption in the function of the thalamus can lead to faulty sensory processing *(see listing for Sensory Processing Disorder)* as well as problems with sleep, cognition and motor control.

TH1 Cells

This type of T cell *(see listing)*, also known as Thymus-Helper 1 cells, plays an important part in cell-mediated immunity and particularly in the adaptive immune system. TH1 cells generate responses to infectious agents such as bacteria and viruses within cells. TH1 cells work with TH2 cells *(see listing)*, but there is often a skewing of the balance of their work towards TH2 cells, which makes it harder to fight off infections from viruses, bacteria and fungal infections. This "TH2 skewing" can be caused by a variety of factors such as yeast overgrowth, stress and the presence of heavy metals in the body such as lead, mercury and aluminum. Children with PANS, neurodevelopmental disorders *(see listing)*, allergies, asthma and autoimmune conditions typically have TH2 skewing.

TH2 Cells

This type of T cell *(see listing)*, also known as Thymus-Helper 2 cells, produces messages to get other immune cells to produce antibodies *(see listing)*, which are used to attack infectious agents such as bacteria and viruses as well as allergens. TH2 cells work outside of infected cells. TH2 cells work with TH1 cells *(see listing)*, but there is often a skewing of the balance of their work towards TH2 cells, which makes it harder to fight off infections from viruses, bacteria and fungal infections. This "TH2 skewing" can be caused by a variety of factors such as yeast overgrowth, stress and the presence of heavy metals in the body such as lead, mercury and aluminum. Children with PANS, neurodevelopmental disorders *(see listing)*, allergies, asthma and autoimmune conditions *(see listing)* typically have TH2 skewing.

TH17 Cells

This type of T cell *(see listing)*, also known as Thymus-Helper 17 cells, plays an important part in cell-mediated immunity, the maintenance of mucosal barriers and pathogen clearance at mucosal surfaces. TH17 cells are pro-inflammatory by virtue of their production of cytokines IL-17 and IL-17F. They recruit neutrophils and macrophages to infected tissues in defense against pathogens.

TH17 cells are implicated in autoimmune and inflammatory disorders.

Tics

Tics are sudden twitches, movements, or behaviors/sounds that happen repeatedly and outside the conscious control of the affected person. Common tics include abnormal and constant eye blinking, frequent shoulder shrugging, or winking. Vocal tics, tongue clicking and throat clearing are also common forms of tics. The same tic can remain constant or can shift to another. A sudden onset of tics often follows a streptococcal or other infection that crosses the blood-brain barrier.

Tomatis Therapy

This is a type of auditory therapy developed by French physician, Alfred Tomatis, an ear, nose and throat specialist. The premise of the therapy is based on the idea that good listeners tune into high-frequency sounds that carry consonants and the meaning of language while inhibiting low-frequency sounds that interfere with this perception. Children with PANS and neurodevelopmental disorders *(see listing)* often have auditory-processing difficulties and may benefit from this type of therapy.

Tourette Syndrome

This neuropsychiatric disorder typically begins in childhood and is characterized by at least one vocal tic *(see listing)* and multiple physical tics. Medical researchers believe that Tourette Syndrome may develop after a streptococcal infection.

Tubulin

These proteins are a component of microtubules, which are structures that are essential for the production, migration and differentiation of neurons. Antibodies *(see listing)* to tubulin are a marker of blood-brain-barrier *(see listing)* dysfunction.

Vibrational Therapy

Vibrational therapy addresses mind-body-spirit imbalances that are often overlooked in Western medicine. Vibrational medicine seeks to balance the "chi" energy in the body. When the body has low "chi" energy, unbalanced vibration or poor energy flow, then sicknesses, imbalances, disease and emotional distress can occur. Examples of vibrational therapy are homeopathy *(see listing)*, essential oils *(see listing)*, acupuncture *(see listing)*, BioSET *(see listing)*, yoga, tai chi *(see listing)*, prayer, reiki, Royal Rife frequencies and bioenergetic medicine *(see listing)*.

Virus

This type of microorganism is smaller than a bacterium and grows and reproduces in other organisms' cells. A virus enters living cells to use their components to keep itself alive and to replicate itself. Viruses cause many common human infections and are also responsible for a number of rare diseases. Children with PANS can often be infected with herpetic viruses such as the Epstein-Barr virus, HHV-6 and cytomegalovirus.

Vision

Vision is not the same thing as eyesight (acuity). Eyesight is the sharpness of the image seen by the eye; vision is the brain's ability to focus on and comprehend that which is seen. Vision processing problems are common in children with PANS as well as neurodevelopmental disorders *(see listing)*, motor delays and vestibular difficulties. A developmental optometrist *(see listing)*, also known as a behavioral optometrist, often uses lenses, prisms and vision therapy to enhance and improve visual function. These interventions can improve a child's academic and behavioral stamina and ability as well as the ability to focus and pay attention.

Vitamin

These organic compounds are derived from food and are essential for normal growth and development. The body cannot make these compounds on its own and thus requires adequate intake.

Children with PANS often have deficiencies of vitamins, such as B vitamins and vitamin D.

Western Blot Test

This controversial immunoblot test for Lyme disease *(see listing)* can detect both IgM *(see listing)* and IgG *(see listing)* antibodies *(see listing)* for specific Lyme-disease proteins. Although Lyme disease is a clinical diagnosis, the U.S. Centers for Disease Control states that at least five IgG bands must be positive in conjunction with a positive enzyme immunoassay (ELISA) for results to be positive for Lyme disease. Because the Western blot test can only test for antibodies to *Borrelia burgdorferi B31*, more Lyme-literate practitioners use the IGeneX test, which can test for more species, and thus has a higher sensitivity for detecting Lyme exposure.

Western Medicine - *see Allopathic Medicine*

Zonulin

This protein regulates the permeability of tight junctions between cells of the wall of the intestine, but it is also found in the brain performing the same duty. Researchers hypothesize that overexpression of it can be involved in increasing blood-brain-barrier *(see listing)* permeability, similar to its role in increasing intestinal permeability *(see listing)*. High zonulin levels are a marker of intestinal permeability, and testing for antibodies to zonulin is a marker of blood-brain-barrier dysfunction.

Zyto

This painless, non-invasive assessment tool is a type of Electro-Dermal Screening *(see listing)* that measures the electrical conductance of the skin to the passage of a small, unfelt electrical current by using a "hand cradle," which is a hand-shaped device on which a hand is placed. It uses the same principle used for lie detectors and biofeedback *(see listing)* devices. It is bundled with software that is programmed to read imbalances in bodily systems. It does not diagnose medical conditions; rather, it is used to support a clinician's assessment.

A SELECTION OF
AVAILABLE RESEARCH

Aldad, T.S., et al. Fetal Radiofrequency Radiation Exposure From 800-1900 Mhz-Rated Cellular Telephones Affects Neurodevelopment and Behavior in Mice. *Sci Rep.* 2012;2:312.

Allen, A.J., et al. Case study: a new infection-triggered, autoimmune subtype of pediatric OCD and Tourette's syndrome. *J Am Acad Child Adolesc Psychiatry.* 1995 Mar;34(3):307-11.

Banks, W.A., et al. Aluminum-induced neurotoxicity: alterations in membrane function at the blood-brain barrier. *Neurosci Biobehav Rev.* 1989 Spring;13(1):47-53.

Baytunca, M.B. [Evaluation of a Neuropsychiatric Disorder: From PANDAS to PANS and CANS]. *Turk Psikiyatri Derg.* 2016 Summer;27(2):0.

Bjarnason, I., et al. Mechanisms of Damage to the Gastrointestinal Tract From Nonsteroidal Anti-Inflammatory Drugs. *Gastroenterology.* 2018 Feb;154(3):500-514.

Boileau, B. A review of obsessive-compulsive disorder in children and adolescents. *Dialogues Clin Neurosci.* 2011;13(4):401-11.

Bora, S.A., et al. Regulation of vitamin D metabolism following disruption of the microbiota using broad spectrum antibiotics. *J Nutr Biochem.* 2018 Jun;56:65-73.

Braniste, V., et al. The gut microbiota influences blood-brain barrier permeability in mice. *Sci Transl Med.* 2014 Nov 19;6(263):263ra158.

Bravo, J.A., et al. Ingestion of Lactobacillus strain regulates emotional behavior and central GABA receptor expression in a mouse via the vagus nerve. *Proc Natl Acad Sci U S A.* 2011 Sep 20;108(38):16050-5.

Brown, K., et al. Pediatric Acute-Onset Neuropsychiatric Syndrome Response to Oral Corticosteroid Bursts: An Observational Study of Patients in an Academic Community-Based PANS Clinic. *J Child Adolesc Psychopharmacol.* 2017 Jul 17.

Brown, K.D., et al. Effect of Early and Prophylactic Nonsteroidal Anti-Inflammatory Drugs on Flare Duration in Pediatric Acute-Onset Neuropsychiatric Syndrome: An Observational Study of Patients Followed by an Academic Community-Based Pediatric Acute-Onset Neuropsychiatric Syndrome Clinic. *J Child Adolesc Psychopharmacol.* 2017 Jul 11.

Butel, M.J., et al. The developing gut microbiota and its consequences for health. *J Dev Orig Health Dis.* 2018 Mar 22:1-8.

Burket, P.R., et al. Pouring fuel on the fire: Th17 cells, the environment, and autoimmunity. *J Clin Invest.* 2015 Jun;125(6):2211-9.

Calaprice, D., et al. A Survey of Pediatric Acute-Onset Neuropsychiatric Syndrome Characteristics and Course. *J Child Adolesc Psychopharmacol.* 2017 Jan 31.

Carpentier, A., et al. Clinical trial of blood-brain barrier disruption by pulsed ultrasound. *Sci Transl Med.* 2016 Jun 15;8(343):343re2.

Chang, K., et al. Clinical evaluation of youth with pediatric acute–onset neuropsychiatric syndrome (PANS): recommendations from the 2013 PANS Consensus Conference. *J Child Adolesc Psychopharmacol.* 2015 Feb;25(1):3-13.

Chiarello, F., et al. An expert opinion on PANDAS/PANS: highlights and controversies. *Int J Psychiatry Clin Pract.* 2017 Jun;21(2):91-98.

Cooperstock, M., et al. Clinical Management of Pediatric Acute-Onset Neuropsychiatric Syndrome: Part III—Treatment and Prevention of Infections. *J Child Adolesc Psychopharmacol.* 2017 Jul, ahead of print.

Cox, C.J., et al. Antineuronal antibodies in a heterogeneous group of youth and young adults with tics and obsessive-compulsive disorder. *J Child Adolesc Psychopharmacol.* 2015 Feb;25(1):76-85.

Dahm, T., et al. Neuroinvasion and Inflammation in Viral Central Nervous System Infections. *Mediators Inflamm.* 2016;2016:8562805.

Dale, R.C. Immune-mediated extrapyramidal movement disorders, including Sydenham chorea. *Handb Clin Neurol.* 2013;112:1235-41.

Dallasta, L.M., et al. Blood-Brain Barrier Tight Junction Disruption in Human Immunodeficiency Virus-1 Encephalitis. *Am J Pathol.* 1999 Dec;155(6):1915-27.

Das, T., et al. Influence of Calcium in Extracellular DNA Mediated Bacterial Aggregation and Biofilm Formation. *PLoS One.* 2014 Mar 20;9(3):e91935.

Dasdaq, S., et al. Effects of 2.4 GHz radiofrequency radiation emitted from Wi-Fi equipment on microRNA expression in brain tissue. *Int J Radiat Biol.* 2015 Jul;91(7):555-61.

DeLong, G.R., et al. Acquired reversible autistic syndrome in acute encephalopathic illness in children. *Arch Neurol.* 1981 Mar;38(3):191-4.

Ding, H., et al. Molecular Pathogenesis of Anti-NMDAR Encephalitis. *Biomed Res Int.* 2015;2015:643409.

Ercan, T.E., et al. Mycoplasma pneumoniae infection and obsessive-compulsive disease: a case report. *J Child Neurol.* 2008 Mar;23(3):338-40.

Ferretti, J.W., et al. Post-Streptococcal Autoimmune Sequelae: Rheumatic Fever and Beyond. *Streptococcus pyogenes: Basic Biology to Clinical Manifestations [Internet].* 2016 Feb 10. Oklahoma City (OK): University of Oklahoma Health Sciences Center.

Fiorentino, M., et al. Blood–brain barrier and intestinal epithelial barrier alterations in autism spectrum disorders. *Molecular Autism.* 2016 Nov 29;7:49.

Frankovich, J., et al. Clinical Management of Pediatric Acute-Onset Neuropsychiatric Syndrome: Part II—Use of Immunomodulatory Therapies. *J Child Adolesc Psychopharmacol.* 2017 Jul

Frankovich, J., et al. Five youth with pediatric acute-onset neuropsychiatric syndrome of differing etiologies. *J Child Adolesc Psychopharmacol.* 2015 Feb;25(1):31-7.

Frankovich, J., et al. Multidisciplinary clinic dedicated to treating youth with pediatric acute-onset neuropsychiatric syndrome: presenting characteristics of the first 47 consecutive patients. *J Child Adolesc Psychopharmacol.* 2015 Feb;25(1):38-47.

Gaughan, T., et al. Rapid Eye Movement Sleep Abnormalities in Children with Pediatric Acute-Onset Neuropsychiatric Syndrome (PANS). *J Clin Sleep Med.* 2016 Jul 15;12(7):1027-32.

Gerardi, D.M., et al. PANDAS and comorbid Kleine-Levin syndrome. *J Child Adolesc Psychopharmacol.* 2015 Feb;25(1):93-8.

Ghaziuddin, M., et al. Brief report: autism and herpes simplex encephalitis. *J Autism Dev Disord.* 1992 Mar;22(1):107-13.

Gherardi, R.K., et al. Biopersistence and Brain Translocation of Aluminum Adjuvants of Vaccines. *Front Neurol.* 2015 Feb 5;6:4.

Gillberg, C. Onset at age 14 of a typical autistic syndrome. A case report of a girl with herpes simplex encephalitis. *J Autism Dev Disord.* 1986 Sep;16(3):369-75.

Greer, M.K., et al. A case study of the cognitive and behavioral deficits of temporal lobe damage in herpes simplex encephalitis. *J Autism Dev Disord.* 1989 Jun;19(2):317-26.

Gulati, G., et al. Anti-NR2 antibodies, blood-brain barrier, and cognitive dysfunction. *Clin Rheumatol.* 2016 Dec;35(12):2989-2997.

Hadjivassiliou, M., et al. Gluten sensitivity: from gut to brain. *Lancet Neurol.* 2010 Mar;9(3):318-30.

Havas, M. Radiation from wireless technology affects the blood, the heart, and the autonomic nervous system. *Rev Environ Health.* 2013;28(2-3):75-84.

Hazlett, H.C., et al. Early brain development in infants at high risk for autism spectrum disorder. *Nature.* 2017 Feb 16;542:348–351.

Herbert, M.R., et al. Autism and EMF? Plausibility of a pathophysiological link part II. *Pathophysiology.* 2013 Jun;20(3):211-34.

Hirai, N., et al. A new infectious encephalopathy syndrome, clinically mild encephalopathy associated with excitotoxicity (MEEX). *J Neurol Sci.* 2017 Sep 15;380:27-30.

Hou, J., et al. Viral interactions with the blood-brain barrier: old dog, new tricks. *Tissue Barriers.* 2016 Jan 28;4(1):e1142492.

Jain, R., et al. The effect of medical treatments on the bacterial microbiome in patients with chronic rhinosinusitis: a pilot study. *Int Forum Allergy Rhinol.* 2018 Mar 8.

Jaspers-Fayer, F., et al. Prevalence of Acute-Onset Subtypes in Pediatric Obsessive-Compulsive Disorder. *J Child Adolesc Psychopharmacol.* 2017 May;27(4):332-341.

Jyonouchi, H., et al. Cytokine profiles by peripheral blood monocytes are associated with changes in behavioral symptoms following immune insults in a subset of ASD subjects: an inflammatory subtype? *J Neuroinflammation.* 2014 Oct 27;11:187.

Kantarcioglu, A.S., et al. Microbiota-Gut-Brain Axis: Yeast Species Isolated from Stool Samples of Children with Suspected or Diagnosed Autism Spectrum Disorders and In Vitro Susceptibility Against Nystatin and Fluconazole. *Mycopathologia.* 2016 Feb;181(1-2):1-7.

Kelly, J.R., et al. Breaking down the barriers: the gut microbiome, intestinal permeability and stress-related psychiatric disorders. *Front Cell Neurosci.* 2015 Oct 14;9:392.

Kim, C., et al. Strep and Urinary Frequency: Is There a Connection? New England Section of the American Urological Association, 75th Annual Meeting. 2006 Sep 28-30.

King, L., et al. Intuition: a critical review of the research and rhetoric. *J Adv Nurs.* 1997 Jul;26(1):194-202.

Kinoshita, M., et al. Targeted delivery of antibodies through the blood-brain barrier by MRI-guided focused ultrasound. *Biochem Biophys Res Commun.* 2006 Feb 24;340(4):1085-90.

Kirvan, C.A., et al. Streptococcal mimicry and antibody-mediated cell signaling in the pathogenesis of Sydenham's chorea. *Autoimmunity.* 2006 Feb;39(1):21-9.

Koffie, R.M., et al. Nanoparticles enhance brain delivery of blood–brain barrier-impermeable probes for in vivo optical and magnetic resonance imaging. *Proc Natl Acad Sci U S A.* 2011 Nov 15;108(46):18837-42.

Kovacevic, M., et al. Use of Intravenous Immunoglobulin in the Treatment of Twelve Youths with Pediatric Autoimmune Neuropsychiatric Disorders Associated with Streptococcal infections. *J Child Adolesc Psychopharmacol.* 2015 Feb;25(1):65-9.

Kreuter, J. Nanoparticles and microparticles for drug and vaccine delivery. *J Anat.* 1996 Dec; 189(Pt 3): 503–505.

Kurlan, R. Tourette's syndrome and 'PANDAS': will the relation bear out? Pediatric autoimmune neuropsychiatric disorders associated with streptococcal infection. *Neurology.* 1998 Jun;50(6):1530-4.

Lancaster, E. The Diagnosis and Treatment of Autoimmune Encephalitis. *J Clin Neurol.* 2016 Jan;12(1):1-13.

Latimer, M.E., et al. Therapeutic plasma apheresis as a treatment for 35 severely ill children and adolescents with pediatric autoimmune neuropsychiatric disorders associated with streptococcal infections. *J Child Adolesc Psychopharmacol.* 2015 Feb;25(1):70-5.

Leclercq, S., et al. Low-dose penicillin in early life induces long-term changes in murine gut microbiota, brain cytokines and behavior. *Nature Communications.* 2017; 8.

Lionetti, E., et al. Gluten Psychosis: Confirmation of a New Clinical Entity. *Nutrients.* 2015 Jul 8;7(7):5532-9.

Mahony, T., et al. Improvement of psychiatric symptoms in youth following resolution of sinusitis. *Int J Pediatr Otorhinolaryngol.* 2017 Jan;92:38-44.

Mahony, T., et al. Palatal Petechiae in the Absence of Group A Streptococcus in Pediatric Patients with Acute-Onset Neuropsychiatric Deterioration: A Cohort Study. *J Child Adolesc Psychopharmacol.* 2017 Apr 7.

Marcello, A., et al. Pediatric Autoimmune Neuropsychiatric Disorders Associated with Streptococcal Infections (PANDAS): An Evolving Concept. *Tremor Other Hyperkinet Mov* (N Y). 2013 Sep 25;3. pii: tre-03-167-4158-7.

Marquet, F., et al. Noninvasive, Transient and Selective Blood-Brain Barrier Opening in Non-Human Primates In Vivo. *PLoS One.* 2011;6(7):e22598.

Mason, R. Expanding Diagnostic Vision with Medical Intuition. *Alternative and Complementary Therapies.* 2009 Mar 19; 6(6).

Mink, J., et al. Acute postinfectious movement and psychiatric disorders in children and adolescents. *J Child Neurol.* 2011 Feb;26(2):214-7.

Muir, K.E., et al. A case report of obsessive-compulsive disorder following acute disseminated encephalomyelitis. *Pediatrics.* 2013 Sep;132(3):e771-4.

Murphy, T.K., et al. Cefdinir for recent-onset pediatric neuropsychiatric disorders: a pilot randomized trial. *J Child Adolesc Psychopharmacol.* 2015 Feb;25(1):57-64.

Murphy, T.K., et al. Characterization of the pediatric acute-onset neuropsychiatric syndrome phenotype. *J Child Adolesc Psychopharmacol.* 2015 Feb;25(1):14-25

Murphy, T.K., et al. A Double-Blind Randomized Placebo-Controlled Pilot Study of Azithromycin in Youth with Acute-Onset Obsessive-Compulsive Disorder. *J Child Adolesc Psychopharmacol.* 2017 Mar 30.

Murphy, T.K., et al. Pediatric acute-onset neuropsychiatric syndrome. *Psychiatr Clin North Am.* 2014 Sep;37(3):353-74.

Nadeau, J.M., et al. A pilot trial of cognitive-behavioral therapy augmentation of antibiotic treatment in youth with pediatric acute-onset neuropsychiatric syndrome-related obsessive-compulsive disorder. *J Child Adolesc Psychopharmacol.* 2015 May;25(4):337-43

Orefici, G., et al. Pediatric Autoimmune Neuropsychiatric Disorders Associated with Streptococcal Infections (PANDAS). *Streptococcus pyogenes: Basic Biology to Clinical Manifestations [Internet].* Oklahoma City (OK): University of Oklahoma Health Sciences Center; 2016-. 2016 Feb 10.

Orlovska, S., et al. Association of Streptococcal Throat Infection With Mental Disorders: Testing Key Aspects of the PANDAS Hypothesis in a Nationwide Study. *JAMA Psychiatry.* 2017 Jul 1;74(7):740-746.

Pall, M.L. Microwave frequency electromagnetic fields (EMFs) produce widespread neuropsychiatric effects including depression. *J Chem Neuroanat.* 2016 Sep;75(Pt B):43-51.

Parker-Athill, E.C., et al. Cytokine correlations in youth with tic disorders. *J Child Adolesc Psychopharmacol.* 2015 Feb;25(1):86-92.

Pearlman, D.M., et al. Anti-basal ganglia antibodies in primary obsessive-compulsive disorder: systematic review and meta-analysis. *Br J Psychiatry.* 2014 Jul;205(1):8-16.

Pihtili, A., et al. Evidence for the Efficacy of a Bioresonance Method in Smoking Cessation: A Pilot Study. *Forsch Komplementmed.* 2014;21(4):239-45.

Plioplys, A.V., et al. Anti-CNS antibodies in childhood neurologic diseases. *Neuropediatrics.* 1989 May;20(2):93-102.

Rawls, W.E., et al. Encephalitis associated with herpes simplex virus. *Ann Intern Med.* 1966 Jan;64(1):104-15.

Sahyouni, R., et al. Effects of concussion on the blood–brain barrier in humans and rodents. *Journal of Concussion.* 2017 Jan 1.

Sai, Y., et al. Clinical diagnosis and treatment of pediatric anti-N-methyl-D-aspartate receptor encephalitis: A single center retrospective study. *Exp Ther Med.* 2018 Aug;16(2):1442-1448.

Samsel, A., et al. Glyphosate, pathways to modern diseases III: Manganese, neurological diseases, and associated pathologies. *Surg Neurol Int.* 2015 Mar 24;6:45.

Shet, A., et al. Immune Response to Group A Streptococcal C5a Peptidase in Children: Implications for Vaccine Development. *J Infect Dis.* 2003 Sep 15;188(6):809-17.

Sifra, S., et al. Treatment of PANDAS and PANS: a systematic review. *Neuroscience & Biobehavioral Reviews.* 2018 Mar;86:51-65.

Singer, H.S., et al. Moving from PANDAS to CANS. *The Journal of Pediatrics.* 2012 May; 160(5):725-731.

Song, Y., et al. Effects of acute exposure to aluminum on blood-brain barrier and the protection of zinc. *Neurosci Lett.* 2008 Nov 7;445(1):42-6.

Spartz, E.J., et al. Course of Neuropsychiatric Symptoms After Introduction and Removal of Nonsteroidal Anti-Inflammatory Drugs: A Pediatric Observational Study. *J Child Adolesc Psychopharmacol.* 2017 Jul 11.

Spindler, K.R., et al. Viral disruption of the blood-brain barrier. *Trends Microbiol.* 2012 Jun;20(6):282-90.

Swedo, S.E., et al. Clinical Presentation of Pediatric Autoimmune Neuropsychiatric Disorders Associated with Streptococcal infections in Research and Community Settings. *J Child Adolesc Psychopharmacol.* 2015 Feb;25(1):26-30

Swedo, S.E., et al. Identification of children with pediatric autoimmune neuropsychiatric disorders associated with streptococcal infections by a marker associated with rheumatic fever. *Am J Psychiatry.* 1997 Jan;154(1):110-2.

Swedo, S.E., et al. Overview of Treatment of Pediatric Acute-Onset Neuropsychiatric Syndrome. *J Child Adolesc Psychopharmacol.* 2017 Jul 19.

Tanaka, S., et al. Autoantibodies against four kinds of neurotransmitter receptors in psychiatric disorders. *J Neuroimmunol.* 2003 Aug;141(1-2):155-64.

Tang, J., et al. Exposure to 900 MHz electromagnetic fields activates the mkp-1/ERK pathway and causes blood-brain barrier damage and cognitive impairment in rats. *Brain Res.* 2015 Mar 19;1601:92-101.

Theoharides, T.C., et al. Neuro-inflammation, blood-brain barrier, seizures and autism. *J Neuroinflammation.* 2011 Nov 30;8:168.

Thienemann M., et al. Clinical Management of Pediatric Acute-Onset Neuropsychiatric Syndrome: Part I-Psychiatric and Behavioral Interventions. *J Child Adolesc Psychopharmacol.* 2017 Jul 19.

Tohidpour, A., et al. Neuroinflammation and Infection: Molecular Mechanisms Associated with Dysfunction of Neurovascular Unit. *Front Cell Infect Microbiol.* 2017 Jun 20;7:276.

Tona, J.T., et al. Impact of PANS and PANDAS Exacerbations on Occupational Performance: A Mixed-Methods Study. *Am J Occup Ther.* 2017 May/Jun;71(3):7103220020P1-7103220020P9.

Toufexis, M.D., et al. Disordered eating and food restrictions in children with PANDAS/PANS. *J Child Adolesc Psychopharmacol.* 2015 Feb;25(1):48-56.

Tuchscherr, L., et al. Staphylococcus aureus phenotype switching: an effective bacterial strategy to escape host immune response and establish a chronic infection. *EMBO Mol Med.* 2011 Mar;3(3):129-41.

Vitaliti, G., et al. A new clinical feature associated with familial early-onset of dystonic-guttural tics: An unusual diagnosis of PANDAS. *J Pediatr Neurosci.* 2014 Jan;9(1):79-81.

Wang, Hsiuying. Anti-NMDA Receptor Encephalitis. *Int J Mol Sci.* 2017 Jan 18;18(1). pii: E193..

Yaddanapudi, K., et al. Passive transfer of streptococcus-induced antibodies reproduces behavioral disturbances in a mouse model of pediatric autoimmune neuropsychiatric disorders associated with streptococcal infection. *Mol Psychiatry.* 2010 Jul;15(7):712-26.

Zong, S., et al. Neuronal Surface Autoantibodies in Neuropsychiatric Disorders: Are There Implications for Depression? *Front Immunol.* 2017 Jul 5;8:752.

RESOURCES

Books:

Blaylock, Russell L. *Excitotoxins: The Taste That Kills.* Health Press, 1996.

Cahalan, Susannah. *Brain on Fire: My Month of Madness.* Simon & Schuster, 2013.

Campbell-McBride, Natasha. *Gut and Psychology Syndrome: Natural Treatment for Autism, Dyspraxia, A.D.D., Dyslexia, A.D.H.D., Depression, Schizophrenia,* 2010.

Chutkin, Robin. *The Microbiome Solution: A Radical New Way to Heal Your Body from the Inside Out.* Avery, 2016.

Giustra-Kozek, Jennifer. *Healing Without Hurting: Treating ADHD, Apraxia and Autism Spectrum Disorders Naturally and Effectively Without Harmful Medication,* 2014.

Hong, Maria Rickert. *Almost Autism. Recovering Children from Sensory Processing Disorder: A Reference for Parents and Practitioners,* 2014.

Lambert, Beth. *A Compromised Generation: The Epidemic of Chronic Illness in America's Children.* Sentient, 2010.

Lemer, Patricia. *Outsmarting Autism,* 2014.

Maloney, Alison Beth. *Saving Sammy: A Mother's Fight to Cure Her Son's OCD.* Broadway Books, 2010.

Weiss, Melanie S. *In a Pickle Over PANDAS.* First Edition Design Publishing, 2015.

Websites:

International OCD Foundation https://iocdf.org/

New England PANS/PANDAS Association http://www.nepans.org/

PANDAS Network http://www.pandasnetwork.org/

Epidemic Answers https://epidemicanswers.org/

Videos:

My Kid Is Not Crazy

PANDAS and PANS with Amy Joy Smith, NP on BetterHealthGuy.com

INDEX

5G antenna 80

A

abdominal pain 15, 163
acidity 72
acid reflux 33, 72, 154, 233
Aconite 96
activity 32, 105, 118, 126, 137, 138,
170, 180, 188, 191, 193
acupressure....104, 145, 153, 160, 193
acupuncture......20, 50, 104, 136, 145,
153, 159, 178, 201
acute symptoms............................. 131
ADD....32, 38, 77, 135, 148, 149, 174,
182, 190, 194
ADHD............................11, 25, 30, 32,
38, 77, 85, 128, 135, 148, 149, 167,
174, 182, 190, 194, 233, 234
adrenal fatigue 197
adrenaline 197
adrenals 61, 76
Advil................................70, 154, 168
AE (autoimmune encephalitis)........12,
13, 23, 24, 43, 57, 67, 71, 107, 116–
121, 123-130, 132-136, 150, 174
aggravants 139, 140, 143
aggression 25, 27, 60, 132
AIDS 28
air filter.. 82
airplane mode 80, 114
alarm clock 80
albumin 189
alcohol 112, 174, 177

alkalinity.. 71
allergies.............. 11, 18, 21, 33, 35, 37,
58, 64, 69, 71, 75, 86, 95, 112, 115,
135, 145, 154, 172, 185
allopathic medicine......7, 44, 64, 116,
146, 170, 185, 202
aluminum............................ 35, 82, 199
Alzheimer's 30, 189, 195
American Academy of Neurology
(AAN) 116
American Association of Integrative
Medicine 134
amino acid 19, 41, 161, 164–166,
181, 183, 194
amoxicillin ....44, 60, 146. *See also*
antibiotics
Anat Baniel method...................... 146
anemia 176
anger 100, 129, 148, 183
anorexia.... 26, 60, 100, 132, 133, 146,
187
antibiotics.......15–17, 19, 29, 31, 34,
44–46, 53, 58, 61, 64–68, 70, 75,
112, 120, 122, 146, 153, 154, 159,
167, 168
antibodies...........28, 29, 33, 40–42, 46,
48, 49, 74, 95, 117, 120, 145, 147,
150, 151, 153, 156–158, 171–175,
183, 185, 187, 189, 193, 194, 196,
199, 200, 202
antibodies to S100-B...............49, 193
antibodies to occludin.................... 49
antibodies to zonulin..............49, 202

antibody testing 49

antigens 30, 41, 48, 147, 156, 158, 171, 172

anti-inflammatory 43, 45, 97, 115, 117, 130, 132, 133

anti-inflammatory diet ... 117, 130, 133

anti-inflammatory interventions .. 132, 133

antimicrobial 76, 97, 98, 112, 115, 122, 131–133, 142, 146

antineuronal antibodies 117, 120

Anti-NMDA Receptor Encephalitis .. 41, 42, 147, 183

anti-parasitics 120

anti-psychotic medications 17

Anti-Streptococcal DNase B (ASDB) 48, 147

Anti-Streptolysin O (ASO) 48, 49, 73, 74, 147, 158, 196

antiviral support 131

anxiety 14, 15, 20, 24–27, 44, 76, 96, 97, 100, 103, 118, 123, 128, 129, 132, 139, 147, 148, 151–153, 156, 159, 160, 162, 164, 170, 173, 177, 180, 183, 184, 187, 190, 192, 193, 197, 198

appetite 57, 194

apple cider vinegar 98

applied kinesiology 50, 51, 61, 62, 92, 148, 153, 180

arsenic 82, 166

ART 50

arthritis 32, 150, 175

artificial colors 87, 195

artificial flavors 87, 195

artificial hormones 135

artificial lights 127

ascorbic acid 99

astatine 143

asthma 11, 35, 85, 134, 135, 152, 154, 159, 167, 168, 171, 173, 177, 199

ASYRA 50, 159

Ativan 44

atopic dermatitis .... 158. *See also* *eczema*

attention 25, 31, 38, 40, 58, 59, 63, 71, 129, 147, 148, 151, 153, 173, 189, 190, 193, 194, 201

attention deficit 148, 193

Auditory Integration Therapy 95, 149

auditory processing 95, 148, 150, 174, 179, 182

Augmentin .... 15, 66, 146. *See also* *antibiotics*

autism 11, 28, 30, 32, 37, 38, 54, 58, 77, 85, 128, 134, 135, 149, 150, 160, 162, 167, 174, 182, 189, 190, 194, 233, 234

auto-antibodies 28, 42, 48, 95, 156

autoimmune disorder 28, 31, 32, 34, 36, 37, 49, 52, 92, 116, 119, 144, 147, 150, 154, 167, 168, 189, 192, 197

Autoimmune Encephalitis panel from Mayo Clinic 117

autoimmune neurology panel 120

autonomic function 105

Avatar 50

azithromycin ...... 60, 66, 147. *See also* *antibiotics*

B

Babesia 16, 18, 47, 53, 97, 108, 111, 175, 184

baby talking .... 26, 64. *See also* *regression*

Bach flower essences 96

bacteria 30–32, 34–37, 45, 49, 55, 56, 67, 90–92, 96, 99, 112, 113, 115, 133, 139, 140, 144, 146, 153, 168, 171, 173, 176, 178, 185, 187, 188, 190, 191, 199

bacterial infection 36, 45, 146, 188

baking soda.. 81
balsam fir oil..................................... 70
banderol 98
Baneil, Anat...................................... 94
balance.........20, 25, 31, 32, 62, 72, 79,
   91, 92, 95, 123, 124, 127, 135, 144,
   149, 156, 170, 176, 190, 192, 196,
   198, 199, 201
barley 42, 166, 167
barley malt.................................42, 166
Bartonella 16, 18, 47, 97, 111, 120,
   175, 184, 187
basal ganglia.........36, 39–41, 150, 151,
   158, 187, 197, 198
B cells......................... 31, 151, 194, 198
bedtime 76, 84, 88, 89
bedwetting.......................... 26, 86, 118
behavior...........7, 11, 13, 14, 24, 26, 30,
   34, 37–39, 44, 45, 68, 86, 94, 100–
   104, 118, 122, 123, 127–129, 138,
   148, 149, 155, 157, 163, 164, 167,
   170, 173, 176, 183–187, 190–192,
   200, 201
behavioral ratings................... 128, 129
behavioral regression........................ 26
behavior therapy...........20, 43, 48, 102,
   103, 129, 132, 155–157,161, 191
benzene 36, 110
berberine..................................98, 168
betaine hydrochloric acid.............. 99
beta lactam antibiotics..................... 44
BiCarb.. 99
Biocidin 98
bioenergetic assessments................. 50
BioEnergetic Medicine.........134, 151,
   201, 234
biofeedback.............102, 105, 106, 127,
   129, 151, 152, 159, 186, 202
biofilm.. 141
bio-individual approach................ 100
biomedical protocol...................... 152
biomedical treatment 60, 100, 152

Biomeridian testing 50, 152
BioRegulation Therapy (BRT)........62,
   102, 105, 106, 152
BioSET 73, 134, 152, 154, 201, 234
biotoxins................................. 111, 180
bipolar disorder 27, 30, 72, 73
bismuth 143
bleach.. 81
blinking.... 26, 64, 65, 200. *See also tic*
Blomberg Rhythmic Movement
   Training......................94, 153, 186
blood-brain barrier 29, 33, 34,
   35, 37, 49, 109, 113, 141, 144, 148,
   151, 153, 160, 166, 179, 185, 187,
   194, 200
blood draw....................................... 66
blood pressure....... 145, 169, 172, 177
bloodwork.....18, 48, 73, 74, 147, 148,
   157, 158, 174, 182, 183
blue light 88, 177
body burden 29, 33, 108, 134
Body Ecology Diet...........88, 153, 154
body image 146
body-mind psychotherapy 101
bodywork.......101, 106, 146, 156, 160
bone broth 42, 166
bouillon 42, 166
Borrelia..... 16, 47, 53, 62, 74, 97, 108,
   175, 184, 202
bowel movements 72, 120
brain-based therapies.....................128
brain fog 123, 180
brain injury.............. 33, 118, 153, 160
brain map.............................. 128, 193
brain stimulation 93
brain waves............ 105, 128, 137, 193
Bravo yogurt............................98, 144
breathing...........92, 122, 123, 145, 151,
   167, 181, 192
breathing difficulties...............92, 167
bromelain.................................69, 99
building materials............................. 80

butyric acid............. 42, 141, 164, 194
B vitamins............................ 19, 92, 202

C
cabinets 80
cadmium 81, 166
Cahalan, Susunnah 41
calcium 110, 141, 193
Campbell-McBride, Natasha 209
Campylobacter................................... 36
cancer 140, 165
Candida albicans............45, 120, 154.
      See also yeast
canola...............................86, 165
CANS (Childhood Acute
      Neuropsychiatric
      Symptoms)......................23, 24, 155
Capanna-Hodge, Roseann........12, 76,
      127, 233
carbohydrates.............66, 86, 175, 195
carcinogens................................31, 164
carnitine 19
carpet.................................. 80, 83, 110
casein..............69, 87, 95, 99, 154, 167
catecholamine................................ 158
cat's claw........................98, 168
cedarwood oil 97
Ceftin.............. 67. See also antibiotics
celiac disease 150, 166
cell phone.............33, 54, 80, 114, 137,
      138, 160
cell phone towers.............................. 33
cellular communication 105, 152
cellular energy................................ 96
cellular toxicity 38
Celtic sea salt.................................... 87
central nervous system............94, 104,
      105, 117, 129, 137, 138, 148–150,
      152, 158, 160, 162, 166, 173, 174,
      182, 186, 190, 193, 194, 197
cephalexin......................65, 66. See also
      antibiotics

cephalosporins................146. *See also*
      antibiotics
cerebellum 144
cerebrospinal fluid.........106, 117, 156
Chamomila...................................... 96
chemical exposure................. 108, 153
Chronic Fatigue Syndrome (CFS)..116
Child Protective Services............... 68
chiropractic 91, 136, 153, 155
chiropractic physicians 91
Chlamydia pneumoniae.........36, 120
chlorine 82
cholera... 122
cholesterol 111, 175
cholesterol sulfate 111
chronic cases......................... 130, 131
cigarette smoke............................... 36
cinnamon oil 68, 70, 161
circadian rhythm.....................84, 178
citrus..............................87, 163, 172
Clean Fifteen 88
clean water........................... 84, 85, 87
clindamycin .... 67, 147. *See also*
      antibiotics
clinginess...................................64, 77
clinical therapies............................ 128
clove oil 68, 70, 161
coaching 128, 129
Cognitive Behavioral Therapy.........20,
      43, 48, 102, 103, 129, 133, 155, 156,
      161, 191
cognitive change.............................. 25
cognitive function 40, 151, 190
colic 58, 71
colloidal silver 62, 76, 98
communication.... 102, 105, 149, 152,
      192
compassion.............................. 123, 124
compromised immune system.......20,
      21, 28, 29, 159, 168, 171, 180
compulsion.......14, 24–26, 73, 75, 100,
      103, 129, 149, 161, 184, 187

compulsive thinking.............14, 26, 75, 103, 129, 149, 161, 184

computer............80, 88, 105, 110, 182

computer games 110

concentration...........95, 148, 149, 157, 176, 179, 181, 182

concussion.................33, 107, 128, 144, 153, 160

consistency 130

constipation.............33, 58, 71, 91, 154, 163, 167, 175

constitutional remedies...........62, 170

convection oven................................ 83

convergence disorder 54, 155, 156

coordination............ 95, 153, 176, 190

copaiba oil...........................68–70, 161

coping skills 102

corded phones................................. 80

cordless phones 33, 80

cordyceps 99

corn..........37, 69, 86, 87, 136, 163, 165, 172, 196

corn syrup... 69

cortical activity 193

cortisol..89, 177

costume jewelry............................... 81

cotton...83, 165

counseling.............. 100, 107, 127, 234

Cowden, William Lee......12, 107, 108, 113, 116

craniosacral therapy.........62, 106, 153, 156, 186

cranium 106, 156

criticism 114

crooked teeth 122

cruciferous vegetables 140

Cunningham, Madeline 48, 156

Cunningham Panel....48, 95, 117, 120, 132, 156, 175

curcumin...............................98, 186

CVID.. 28

cysteine...........................166, 179, 181

cytokine......................32, 34, 108, 199

cytomegalovirus (CMV).....36, 63, 64, 66, 73, 201

D

dairy.............87, 95, 120, 136, 154, 163, 165, 172, 196

dehumidifier..................................... 80

dementia 116

depression................25, 26, 30, 53, 60, 61, 75, 92, 100, 129, 139, 156, 157, 175, 183, 187, 192, 194, 234

deterioration.....................25, 132, 174

detoxification......19, 45, 53, 54, 62, 84, 91, 96, 97, 99, 120, 124, 127, 131, 140–142, 159, 166, 170, 171, 174, 175, 178, 179, 181, 184, 188, 191

detoxification pathways........127, 140, 141

developmental delays........11, 86, 176, 184, 190

developmental milestones........38, 58

developmental optometrist....94, 156, 157, 196, 201

developmental physician 94

developmental regression.............. 26

diagnosis 13, 15, 23, 24, 28, 38, 41, 49, 64, 94, 107, 115, 119, 121, 122, 132, 147–150, 156, 175, 182, 183, 191, 194, 202

Diagnostic and Statistical Manual (DSM) 128

Dialectical Behavior Therapy (DBT).. 102, 103, 157

diaper rash 58, 71

diarrhea.................58, 71, 91, 122, 154, 163, 167

die-off reaction 125

diet...............31, 38, 44, 53, 56, 66, 69, 76, 84–92, 117, 118, 120, 121, 123, 130, 131, 133, 135, 141, 143, 153, 154, 165–168, 177, 178, 183, 186,

188, 195, 196, 197
diet modification 118, 122, 131
digestive aids 99
digestive enzymes.....................99, 154
digestive function 131
Dirty Dozen 88
disinfectants 81
distraction.......................................128
DNA................................164, 165, 179
DNase B.................48, 49, 67, 132, 147,
157, 158
Doctors Data 96
dopamine...............40, 41, 48, 149, 151,
156, 158, 183
dopamine D1 receptor (DRD1)........48,
156
dopamine D2L receptor (DRD2L)......
48, 156
dopamine receptors....40, 41, 151, 158
downtime....................................55, 76
DPP-IV 99
dread.. 147
drug-free approach 92
dryer sheets 81
duodenum.. 112
dyscalculia....................................... 174
dysgraphia....................................... 174
dyslexia 128, 158, 174, 182

E
ear infection 58, 71
eczema.... 33, 35, 58, 71, 86, 134, 135,
158, 159, 177
educational assessments 191
electroencephalography (EEG)....117,
128, 193
eggs...............................87, 88, 163, 196
electroacupuncture......... 50, 152, 159
electro-dermal screening 74
electromagnetic radiation 33, 80
electronic appliance......................... 80
electronic device............................... 80

EMFs (ElectroMagnetic Fields).....33,
54, 105, 110, 111, 113, 114, 123, 124,
126, 127, 136, 153, 160, 192, 197
emotional acupressure 104
emotional brain 104, 162
emotional environment 114
Emotional Freedom Technique
(EFT)...99, 102, 104, 129, 160, 198
emotional function 39, 40, 151
emotional lability.............. 25, 26, 129
emotional stress..............26, 35, 53, 54,
104, 113, 177, 186, 197
emotional trauma.....35, 106, 113, 121
encephalopathy.........12, 18, 24, 27, 28,
30, 35, 36, 41, 42, 43, 67, 116–121,
127, 132, 133, 147, 150, 160, 161,
174, 183
endocrine disruptors 31, 164
endorphins....................................... 106
endoscopy 71
energetic testing 112
energy medicine.....102, 151, 162, 169,
170, 178
energy meridians............................ 104
energy psychotherapy................... 102
energy work............................ 101, 102
enthromycin.....67. See also antibiotics
enuresis 25
environment................. 11, 12, 25, 32,
35, 36, 44, 45, 52, 54, 76, 80, 88, 89,
107–111, 113, 114, 118, 123, 130,
133, 136, 149, 150, 163–166, 170,
174, 175, 179, 180, 182, 187
environmental toxins.........36, 80, 149,
150, 163, 164, 174, 175, 179, 182
Environmental Working Group.....84,
88
enzyme production....................... 111
enzyme therapy 152, 153
Epidemic Answers...........8, 11, 12, 57,
75, 76, 79, 86, 90, 134, 233
epigenetic vulnerabilities............... 29

epinephrine 145, 172, 183, 197
Epstein-Barr virus (EBV).....43, 47, 64, 73, 77, 97, 184, 201
Erythromycin...........................146. *See also antibiotics*
essential fatty acids 53, 88, 90, 93
essential oils...... 68, 69, 81, 82, 97, 98, 161, 201
etiology............................. 117
excitotoxicity.....41, 42, 161, 166, 183
executive functioning........... 128, 129
exercise............20, 55, 84, 93, 127, 155, 181, 192
exhaustion............................. 62
Exposure Therapy (ERP).......102, 103, 129, 161
eyelash pulling 26
eye movement......40, 59, 99, 102, 103, 151, 162
Eye Movement Desensitization and Reprocessing (EMDR).........59, 99, 102, 103, 129, 162, 186, 234
eyes, dilated................64, 66
eyesight.............................94, 157, 201

F
fabric softener 81
"failure to thrive" 179, 184
family constellations............. 102, 162
family therapy 70
family time..................................... 123
fan...................................73, 75, 80, 160
farmer's market.............................. 143
farming practices............................ 126
fast foods...................................... 85
fatigue..........7, 118, 157, 160, 177–180, 188, 195, 197
fats................85, 87, 123, 141, 144, 175, 194, 195
fear.....14, 58, 61, 68, 70, 96, 104, 139, 147, 184
fear of eating.................................... 14

fermentation...................................... 88
fermented foods 88, 98
"fight or flight" 137, 148, 190, 197
flame retardants.............................. 82
flares................18, 33, 62, 70, 124, 129
flavors 87, 195
fluorescent light bulbs..................... 82
fluoride 82, 149
focus..........47, 56, 93–95, 97, 105, 115, 127, 128, 148, 149, 157, 158, 167, 170, 179, 182, 189, 201
folate 19, 179, 180
folic acid 69, 179
food additives.............................42, 166
food allergies...............33, 86, 115, 171, 185, 186
food intolerance........................58, 154
food restriction 25, 26, 146
food rules 84, 85
food sensitivities.......86, 95, 149, 150, 163, 166, 167, 182, 196
food supply 126
formaldehyde 36, 82, 110
frankincense oil 68, 70, 97, 161
free radical 90, 181, 186
fresh air............................... 55, 83, 123
Frid, Elena..............................12, 116
frontal cortex...................34, 109, 113
Fukushima 143
functional dentist 122, 181
functional lab testing..................... 131
functional medicine..........61, 90, 152, 153, 163
functional nutrition 131
fungi................30, 35, 45, 55, 153, 173, 176, 180, 199
furnishings....................................... 80

G
GABA (gamma-aminobutyric acid)......42, 76, 148, 164, 167, 183, 186

GAD65-receptor antibodies 117
garlic 98
gastroenterologist 71
gastrointestinal pain 26, 118
gastrointestinal tract.................31, 32, 120, 122, 154, 168, 171, 176, 178, 183, 194
Gates, Donna...........................88, 153
gelatin 42, 166
genetic mutation.......21, 149, 164, 179
genetic testing................................ 128
Genova Diagnostics........................ 96
germ fears 70
Gervanius...................................... 96
glass... 82
glue.. 14, 15, 80
glutamate....................41, 42, 147, 161, 164–167, 183, 186
glutamic acid 164, 166
glutathione.....141, 166, 180, 181, 186
glutathione pathway 141
gluten.............37, 66, 69, 70, 87, 95, 99, 120, 153, 163, 166–168, 172, 196
gluten-free/casein free diet (GFCF) .. 167
glycine...............41, 161, 166, 183, 188
glyphosate..........36, 37, 154, 166, 168
GMOs........ 85, 86, 126, 165, 168, 196
grapefruit seed extract 98
Great Plain Laboratories................ 96
gross motor skills 176
grounding................. 76, 110, 111, 167
growth delays 179, 184
gut bacteria.............32, 34, 37, 56, 92
gut-brain connection..................... 112
gut dysbiosis........................29, 38, 45, 53, 90–92, 96, 121, 135, 146, 149, 152–154, 158, 163, 167, 168, 171, 174, 176, 178, 181–184, 188, 191, 194, 196
gut permeability..............29, 32, 34, 37, 112, 115, 173, 174

H

Hahnemann, Samuel 62
hair pulling 26, 73
hallucinations.............................27, 192
hand flapping 149
hand-washing............... 66. *See also* tic
handwriting...15, 20, 27, 132, 174, 187
hardwiring 80
harmonic frequencies.................... 152
headaches......15, 65, 67, 74, 101, 147, 148, 160, 167, 173, 180, 181, 195
head banging.................................... 27
head-circumference percentile..... 28, 161
head injury.......................33, 107, 108
head pain..15, 16, 64–67, 74, 101, 147, 148, 160, 163, 167, 169, 173, 180, 181, 195
head turning................. 64. *See also* tic
healing.............8, 11, 12, 14, 32, 56, 58, 61–63, 69, 70, 75, 77, 79, 84, 85, 89, 91, 95, 99, 100, 101, 105, 106, 114, 118, 121, 123, 124, 127, 130, 131, 133, 134, 136, 137, 142, 153, 162, 168, 169, 172, 181, 183, 188, 192, 198
healing environment....114, 118, 123, 130, 133
health coach 8, 74, 75, 89, 90
hearing........................60, 95, 149, 193
heart palpitations 160
heart rate........................105, 151, 197
heavy metals...........31, 36, 52, 81, 164, 166, 173, 181, 199
hepatitis B 36
herbal medicine..........61, 98, 112, 114, 120, 133, 168, 181
herbal tinctures.........................76, 112
herpes 36, 47
herpetic viruses 73, 150, 175, 201
Herxheimer reaction 125, 168
HHV-6.......................................73, 201

Himalayan salt 76, 87
histamine 143, 169, 175, 177, 183
histamine diet 143, 177
hives 21, 145
holistic......................50, 86, 90, 91, 101,
    129, 130, 134, 136, 169, 172, 181,
    233, 234
homeopaths................................91, 96
homeopathy......62, 76, 130, 153, 169,
    170, 181, 201
homeostasis............................ 101, 135
homeschooling 130
homotoxicologist.......................73, 97
hope 11, 12, 14, 17, 21, 57, 66, 116,
    133, 233
hormone imbalances 127
hormones..........88, 127, 135, 158, 165,
    170, 175, 177, 197
Huntington's......................40, 138, 151
hydration.. 55
hydrogenated oils 86
hydrolyzed vegetable protein...........42,
    166
hyperactivity.....25, 27, 148, 149, 153,
    181, 189
hypnosis 102, 104, 129, 170
hypothalamus................................144
hypnotherapy 104, 170, 234

I
IgA........................... 120, 145, 163, 171
IgE 145, 163, 171, 172
IGeneX 175, 202
IgG............ 74, 120, 145, 163, 172, 202
IgM 74, 120, 145, 163, 172, 202
immune dysregulation 38, 92, 134,
    135, 146, 148–150, 152, 158, 159,
    163, 168, 170, 171, 174, 178, 180,
    181, 182, 187, 194
immune-modulating therapy.......117
immune system..... 18–20, 28–32, 35,
    37, 39, 40–43, 45, 46, 53, 58, 61,
    62, 67, 68, 81, 107, 108, 110–112,
    117, 120, 121, 124, 127, 132, 134,
    138, 139, 144, 147, 150, 151, 153,
    154, 159, 161, 168, 170–173, 176,
    178, 180, 198, 199
immunoglobulin levels..................132
immunotherapy..............................174
impulsive behavior........................148
Independent Physicians of New York
    (IDNY)......................................116
individualized approach................133
infection........15, 18, 19, 21, 24, 26, 28,
    29, 32, 33, 35, 36, 40, 44–52, 55,
    58, 60, 63, 64, 67, 69, 71, 74–76,
    97, 98, 116, 117, 119–121, 126,
    132, 138, 144, 146–148, 150, 151,
    153–157, 160, 166, 167, 172, 173,
    175–177, 180, 184, 186–188, 196,
    197, 199–201
inflammation.................16, 19, 27, 28,
    30, 32, 33, 35, 37, 42, 44, 45, 67, 69,
    89, 97, 98, 115, 117, 119–124, 126,
    127, 132, 134, 135, 146, 147, 149,
    150, 152, 154, 158, 160, 163, 167,
    174, 176, 177, 179, 181, 182, 184,
    186, 188, 193, 194, 197
Influenza 47
infrared light....................................114
injectable adjuvants 35, 153
injectable medical products 35
insecticides 36
insomnia..173
insulation 80
integrative clinicians....28, 85, 86, 90,
    116
integrative medicine........46, 134, 153,
    172
interferon 32
interleukins.. 32
International and American
    Association of Clinical
    Nutritionists 136

International Foundation of Health and Nutrition 136
International Lyme and Associated Diseases Society (ILADS) 116
intuition 51, 52, 63
iodine 93, 113, 143, 178
Iodoral 113
iron 53, 73, 82, 90, 93, 176
irritability 25, 163, 181
itching 169
IVIG (intravenous immunoglobulin) 16, 19, 43, 46, 70, 117, 121, 122, 146, 171, 173

J

jerking .... 26. *See also tic*
jin shin jyutsu 99, 173, 186
joint pain 126
junk food 55

K

K+ channel receptor antibodies ... 117, 174
Katz, Sandor 88
kefir 88, 98
kinesiology .... 50, 51, 61, 62, 92, 148, 153, 180, 193. *See also muscle testing*
kinetic energy 104
Klonopin 44
Kobliner, Victoria 12, 131

L

lab tests 49, 51, 64–66, 117, 120, 128, 132
lactose intolerance 154
language 95, 149, 158, 179, 200
latching on 71
laundry soap 81
lavender oil 70, 97
lead 29, 32–35, 37, 45, 81, 92, 122, 124, 126, 145, 149,

158, 159, 161, 164, 166, 168, 169, 171, 176, 178, 179, 184, 198, 199
leafy greens 88
leaky brain 34, 37
leaky gut 29, 32, 34, 37, 112, 115, 173, 174
learning 8, 40, 60, 89, 94, 100, 105, 128, 151, 161, 166, 174, 176, 182, 190, 191, 194
learning disability 128, 174, 182, 190, 194
Lemer, Patricia 12, 54
lemon 81
Lexapro 44
Licensed Clinical Social Worker (LCSW) 192
Licensed Marriage and Family Therapist (LMFT) 192
Licensed Professional Counselor (LPC) 127, 192, 233
life force energy 106
lifestyle changes 12, 38, 44, 89, 91, 117, 130, 135, 136, 155, 233
linoleum 80
Lipman, Frank 84
listening therapy 95, 174
Listerine 69
liver 45, 88, 122, 141, 154, 159, 169, 174, 175, 188
love 23, 54, 55, 89, 90, 123
low blood sugar 74, 166
Lugol's iodine 113
Lyme disease 16, 24, 61, 73, 74, 76, 175, 180, 202
lymphatic tissue 138
lymphocytes 31, 151, 198
lysoganglioside GM1 ...... 48, 156, 175

M

Maalox 71
magic bullet 109
magnesium 53, 90, 93, 110, 148, 178

malabsorption.............................96, 176
malnutrition 176
manganese...36
mannose-binding lectin........ 120, 176
Manuka honey 98
mast-cell activation..................35, 177
mathematics disabilities........ 109, 174
math skills................ 27, 109, 174, 187
mattresses.. 82
Mayo Clinic 117
measles.. 36
medical intuitives.......................51, 52
Medical Medium............................. 73
medicinal mushrooms..................... 99
meditation 99, 186, 192
melatonin................. 88, 177, 178, 197
memory deficit................................. 25
memory, short-term 20, 33, 198
mercury.................... 82, 150, 166, 199
meridians 50, 104, 145, 152, 178
metabolic issues............................... 47
metabolism...........47, 58, 96, 110, 152,
    162, 178
methylfolate...................................... 69
microbes........... 16, 28, 30, 32, 34, 40,
    41, 47, 52, 53, 56, 90, 108, 109, 111,
    113, 114, 136, 142, 171, 178, 183
microbiome 31, 45, 47, 88, 92, 148,
    150, 159, 168, 178, 182, 190
microbiota 34, 178
microwave ovens 33
milk 144, 154, 167
mind-altering medication.............. 68
minerals...........61, 72, 87, 93, 169, 178,
    184, 196
mistake...........115, 118, 124, 125, 130,
    133, 150, 179
mitochondrial dysfunction......19, 38,
    96, 179, 188
mold..... 31, 36, 55, 81, 107, 108–110,
    119, 123, 136, 138–140, 146, 180
molecular mimicry....40, 41, 158, 179

mood..............7, 24, 26, 30, 44, 62, 67,
    74, 77, 86, 101, 139, 154, 156, 164,
    167, 168, 176, 183, 185, 186, 190,
    192, 194, 197
mood swings 26, 74, 77
Moorcroft, Tom................... 6, 12, 119
motor abnormalities........................ 25
motor cortex........................... 113, 179
motor development 38, 190
motor function.................. 20, 39, 114
motor movement.....................39, 158
Motrin 65, 68, 69, 154, 168
mouth breathing............................122
movement.....................35, 36, 39, 40,
    55, 59, 72, 84, 93, 94, 99, 102, 103,
    120, 123, 144, 150, 151, 153, 158,
    162, 176, 179, 186, 187, 190, 192,
    194, 197, 198, 200
movement disorder.....36, 39, 40, 151
MRI 16, 117
MSG (monosodium glutamate).....42,
    166
MTHFR....19, 21, 53, 69, 140, 165, 179
mumps.. 36
muscle contraction 123
muscle testing..........50, 51, 61, 62, 92,
    139, 141, 148, 153, 180, 193
musculoskeletal system........ 155, 186
Masgutova Method..........94, 176, 186,
    190
myasthenia gravis...........................138
Mycoplasma pneunomiae...............77
mycotoxin...........31, 36, 108, 109, 138,
    139, 180
Mylanta 71
myofunctional therapist....... 122, 181
myrrh oil 70

N
N-acetylcysteine (NAC)..........99, 181
nasal surgery.....................................67

naso-gastric feeding support..........16, 17, 19

natural flavors 42, 87, 166, 195

naturopath 61, 62, 76, 91, 159, 181

nausea 148, 169, 195

negative emotions 104

negative self-talk............................100

negative thoughts 104, 170

neurocognitive assessment...........117

neurocognitive functioning..........128

neurofeedback..........76, 102, 105, 127, 129, 182, 183, 186, 233, 234

neuroinflammation........30, 33, 35, 38, 47, 48, 94, 95

neurologist.....16, 18, 65, 68, 116, 182

neuromovement 94

neuropsychiatric symptoms............24, 25, 41, 48, 117, 119, 125, 131, 133, 155, 158, 187

neuroscience 96, 128

Neurosciences Laboratory 96

neurotransmitter 40, 42, 96, 115, 149, 150, 158, 161, 165, 169, 170, 182, 183, 194

neurotypical child..................119, 125, 131, 133

New England PANS/PANDAS Association 91

niacin 92

night sweats.....................................122

nitric oxide.......................................114

NMDA receptor (N-methyl-D-aspartate receptor).............41, 117, 161, 183

noise sensitivity 60, 62

non-laboratory methods of testing..50

non-stick cookware........................ 82

norepinephrine 183

nosode remedies......................62, 170

NSAIDs (nonsteroidal anti-inflammatory drugs)......43, 45, 46

numbness.. 15

nurse practitioners...........................91

NutrEval 96

nutrient testing 92

nutrient therapy...............................150

nutrition............17, 19, 54, 55, 62, 76, 85, 89, 92, 131, 134, 136, 153, 170, 176, 183, 184, 234

nutritional deficiencies........19, 29, 42, 45, 53, 64, 90, 92, 93, 96, 110, 111, 130, 134, 146, 148, 149, 152, 153, 158, 168, 174, 176, 181, 182, 184, 194, 196

nutritionist....19, 73, 74, 85, 134, 136, 234

nuts......................37, 87, 163, 171, 172

O

oats 37, 87, 166, 167

obesity...126

obsession..........60, 103, 129, 149, 161, 184

occipital lobe 109, 113, 114, 185

occludin.....................................49, 185

occupational therapy.........20, 94, 176, 190

OCD (Obsessive-Compulsive Disorder) 14, 15, 20, 24–27, 41, 64, 96, 100, 103, 125, 129, 132, 158, 183, 184, 187, 192, 234

ODD (Oppositional Defiant Disorder) 24, 26, 185, 187

oil.....68–70, 76, 81, 82, 86–88, 97, 98, 161, 165, 168, 195, 201

olive leaf 65, 69, 98, 168

omega fatty acids............... 65, 69, 186

open bites...122

oppositional behavior...................... 25

oral allergy syndrome.............21, 185

oregano oil 98, 168

organic cause...................................116

organic food 62, 85

organizational skills 95, 182

oro-facial structural abnormalities.... 122, 181
osteopathic physician 90, 122, 181
osteopathy.............................. 181, 185
outdoor environments 29, 89, 111
oxidative stress................. 90, 166, 186
oxygen.................................. 122, 181

P

pain...... 15, 16, 19, 26, 59, 61, 64, 101, 105, 106, 118, 126, 145, 151, 159, 163, 169, 170, 173, 190, 192, 195
pain reduction................................ 105
paint.............................80, 81, 110, 142
PANDAS (Pediatric Autoimmune Neuropsychiatric Disorders Associated with Streptococcal Infections)............7, 8, 12, 13, 15, 16, 19, 20, 23, 24, 30, 32, 36, 40, 44–46, 57, 60, 61, 63, 68, 71, 73, 74, 75, 77, 91, 107, 108–111, 113–118, 120, 121, 123–126, 128–136, 146, 166, 187, 188, 234
PANDAS Network 91
panic...............................103, 147, 162
PANS (Pediatric Acute-onset Neuropsychiatric Syndrome)......7, 8, 12–14, 16, 19, 23–25, 27–41, 43–49, 51, 52, 54, 56, 57, 63, 71, 74, 75, 77, 79, 80, 84–86, 91–93, 95, 100–102, 107–111–118, 120, 121, 123–126, 128–137, 139, 144, 146–190, 192–202
PANS/PANDAS-literate practitioner 131
papaya..................................... 99
parasites 30, 168, 171, 178
parasympathetic nervous system....... 137, 138, 160, 186, 197
parietal lobe...................113, 114, 187
Parkinson's.....................30, 36, 40, 151
pathogen........29, 30, 33, 43, 44, 47, 50, 74, 97, 99, 138, 139, 141, 147, 153, 163, 171, 172, 179, 184, 186, 188, 191, 199
pathophysiology 38
patience 61, 100, 125, 130
Paxil...................................... 44
Peace and Calming oil 70
Pediasure.................................72
pediatrician........13, 15, 60, 64, 68, 71, 73, 76, 126
PEMF....102, 105, 106, 129, 152, 186, 192
penicillin 34, 44, 146
perceived evaluation...................... 113
perfect storm................................ 52
perfume............................... 82
persistence 130
personality changes...................... 187
pest-control products..................... 82
pesticides.....30, 36, 37, 52, 54, 58, 88, 126, 135, 140, 143, 196
pharmaceutical medications....44, 45, 76, 83, 146, 152, 168
phase-one detoxification.......141, 175, 188
phase-two detoxification.......141, 175, 188
phase-three detoxification....141, 175, 188
pH changes 176
phenols................................ 87
phobias 27, 104
phosphatidylserine.......... 69, 188, 189
phospholipid 141, 188, 189
photonic enhanced uptake 114
physical activity 118, 137
physical exam.............................. 120
physician assistants....................... 91
picky eating................. 118, 184, 196
pineal gland 177
PITAND (Pediatric Infection Triggered Autoimmune

Neuropsychiatric Disorders)........13, 23, 24, 187, 188
plasma......................43, 46, 175, 189
plasmapheresis........................43, 189
plastic...............................81, 82
Pollan, Michael 84
pollution............................. 177
polysorbate 80................................. 35
poor eating.....21. *See also picky eating*
Post-Traumatic Stress Disorder (PTSD).............. 101, 162, 189, 190
potassium......................................174
powerlines................................. 33
prayer...........................99, 201
preservatives.................... 87, 163, 195
Prevacid.............................. 72
prevention...11, 12, 103, 127, 129, 161
Price Pottenger Nutritional Foundation................................ 136
primitive reflexes...93, 148–150, 153, 176, 182, 190, 197
probiotics........62, 68, 69, 98, 144, 188, 190, 191
procedural learning......... 40, 151, 191
processed foods............36, 42, 85, 120, 134, 165, 166, 195
projectile vomit...........................58, 71
propolis 98
protein...........37, 42, 46, 48, 49, 74, 85, 87, 150, 154, 157, 166, 167, 171, 174, 176, 179, 185, 193, 200, 202
proteolytic enzymes......................... 99
Prozac................................. 44
psychiatric drug............................115
psychiatric symptoms.........13, 38, 61, 115, 125, 131
psychiatrist 15, 191
psychoactive medication 132
psychoeducation............103, 129, 161
psychological acupressure............ 104
psychologist............15, 68, 73, 76, 100, 102, 127, 136, 191, 233, 234

psychosis..........41, 147, 187, 191, 192
psychotherapist................62, 192, 234
psychotherapy 15, 59, 62, 68, 73, 76, 100–103, 127, 129, 136, 155, 157, 162, 191, 192, 233, 234
psychotropic medications.........18, 48, 119, 156
Pulsed Electromagnetic Field Therapy (PEMF) 102, 105, 106, 129, 152, 186, 192

Q
QBC.............................. 69
QEEG (Quantitative Electroenceph-alography) 128, 129, 193
Qest4................................. 50
qi gong.............................99, 186, 192
Quantum Reflex Analysis.....134, 193, 234
quercetin 69

R
rabbit hole............................. 14
radiation......................33, 80, 143, 164
radio frequency............................. 144
radon................................. 81
rage....15, 17, 21, 26, 39, 74, 100, 129, 157
Rapp, Doris........................ 86
rashes...................... 126, 163, 169, 175
rational brain......................... 104, 162
reactivation....................................... 33
reading.... 95, 109, 128, 153, 155, 158, 174, 179
reading disabilities 128
RealSalt............................... 87
recovery.........18, 21, 68, 77, 123, 193
red dye................................. 69
red flags 20
refrigerator.....................80, 160
regression of behavior 118
reiki 62, 102, 106, 129, 201, 234

reishi 99
relapse 34, 46
relaxation techniques 104
repetitive behavior 184
resilience 55, 140
restrictive eating 178, 187
retained primitive reflexes 93, 149,
150, 176, 182, 190
rheumatic fever 67, 197
rhythmic movement 94, 153, 186,
190
Robert Wood Johnson Medical
School Alumni Association 116
rocking 57, 59, 149
root causes 3, 9, 38, 52, 56, 89, 90,
131, 146, 149, 150, 152, 158, 163,
164, 170, 174, 181, 182, 194
Round-up 36, 154, 166, 168
rye 166, 167

S
salicylates 87
saline 189
salt foot baths 19
samento 98, 168
sandalwood oil 97
school performance 25, 132
SCID 28, 194
scratch test 145
screen time 76, 127
seaweed 42, 166
sedentary lifestyle 126
seizure 27, 42, 147, 150, 160,
161, 180, 183
selenium 93
self-stimulating behavior 149
sensory integration 38
sensory issues 20, 187
Sensory Processing Disorder 32,
38, 76, 77, 167, 174, 182, 187, 190,
193, 194, 197, 198, 233
separation anxiety 26

serotonin 139, 183, 194
Shapiro, Francine 103, 162
shingles 73
short-chain fatty acid 141, 194
shoulder shrugging .... 26, 64, 200.
See also tic
siding 80
silent reflux 71
single-nucleotide polymorphism
(SNP) 164, 179
sinus infection 63, 64, 67, 75, 167
skin crawling 123
skin temperature 105, 151
sleep 16, 21, 25, 26, 53–55, 58,
60, 65, 66, 69, 71, 74, 80, 84, 88,
111, 123, 124, 127, 130, 132, 147,
156, 157, 160, 176–178, 180, 181,
187, 192, 194, 197, 198
sleep apnea 54, 181
sleep disturbance 25, 127, 132,
181, 187
sleep sanctuary 124
sleep schedule 127
slow-wave sleep 127
small intestine 112, 113, 166, 188
smart meters 33, 54, 80, 114, 160
smartphones 80, 88
socialization 179
social stressors 121
social withdrawal 194
soft signs 20, 21, 33, 58, 71
solvents 36
somatic symptoms 25, 74, 195
Sound Stimulation 95, 195
soy ...42, 86, 87, 136, 163, 166, 172, 196
soy protein isolate 42, 166
soy sauce 42, 166
SPECT scan 117, 195
speech 38, 64, 95, 109, 153, 179,
181, 192, 197
speech delay 181
speech development 38

spirituality.............................. 101, 102
SSRIs...................................... 139
stainless steel................................. 82
Standard American Diet............53, 92, 154, 168, 178, 183, 186, 195, 197
standard of care 75
statistics... 27
steroids 43, 45, 46, 159
Stetzer dirty electricity filters 76
stevia..98, 168
Still, A.T.. 122
stimming... 149
stomach................. 17, 59, 74, 112, 113
stomach aches.................................. 74
Stone, Lauren 6, 12, 134, 234
strabismus...................................54, 196
Strep.............15, 16, 18, 24, 28, 40, 41, 48, 49, 53, 58–64, 66–68, 73, 74, 76, 77, 108, 111, 132, 135, 147, 155, 158, 166, 187, 196
Strep titer 64, 66, 67, 132, 196
stress 8, 11, 26, 29, 32, 35, 45, 50, 53–56, 59, 61, 62, 73, 75, 76, 79, 80, 84, 89, 90, 99, 101, 103–107, 113, 121, 124, 126, 127, 128, 129, 130, 132, 147, 151, 153, 154, 160, 162, 164, 166, 168, 170, 176–178, 184–186, 189, 193, 197, 199
stress reduction 105, 106, 130
stress-reduction therapies............ 101
stroke 28
structural abnormalities....... 122, 181
structural changes.......................... 121
subconscious..........101, 104, 105, 129, 170, 182
sudden onset......24, 126, 131, 137, 200
sugar................................59, 66, 69, 70, 74, 85, 86, 110, 120, 134, 154, 165, 166, 174–176, 197
suicide............................... 44, 100, 157
sulfation pathway 141

sulfur..140
sun exposure 54, 83, 84
sunglasses... 89
sunlight.... 29, 54, 54, 83, 84, 110, 177
sunscreen 83, 84, 89, 111
supplements 19, 62, 65, 69, 70, 76, 98, 130, 131, 133, 141, 164, 170, 180, 181, 184, 186, 188, 196
support 11, 12, 16, 19, 43, 47, 51, 55, 61, 62, 65, 69, 75, 76, 84, 85, 89, 91, 98–102, 120, 121, 123, 124, 128–134, 140, 142, 158, 159, 168, 169, 183, 192, 202
support groups...........................91, 133
suppressed emotions............ 104, 170
Swedo, Sue.................................24, 132
Sydenham chorea............ 25, 132, 197
sympathetic nervous system........105, 137, 138, 148, 160, 190, 197

T
tablets 80, 88, 112, 113, 196
tai chi 99, 186, 198, 201
talk therapy............. 101, 129, 191, 192
tantrums....................................26, 60
tapping..... 99, 102, 104, 129, 160, 198
task completion 128
T cells.................31, 46, 151, 194, 198
tea tree oil 81, 97
technology 13, 106, 126, 142, 152
Teflon.. 82
temporal lobe.................33, 109, 198
terrain.............................111, 135, 142
TH1 cells............................. 144, 199
TH2 cells 144, 199
TH17 cells......138, 144, 180, 199, 200
thalamus..........................40, 150, 198
Theoharides, Theo.......................... 35
Thieves oil 97
throat clearing......64, 200. *See also tic*
throat culture 49
throat pain 126

thumb sucking 64

thrush 154

thyme oil 70, 81, 97, 168

thyroid 19, 143, 178

tic........7, 15, 19, 24, 26, 36, 38–41, 64,
65, 67, 68, 75, 118, 122, 129, 158,
183, 187, 200

tick-borne illnesses 19, 21

tingling 15

tipping point................................32, 55

tobacco 83

toluene... 110

Tomatis therapy........................95, 200

tomatoes...................................42, 166

tongue clicking........... 200. *See also tic*

tongue tie 71, 181

tonsillectomy................ 60, 65,–67, 75

tonsillitis.. 67

total load of stressors.......4, 29, 54, 55,
80, 134, 154, 164

total load syndrome 134

Tourette..........27, 36, 64, 68, 132, 200

toxic body burden 29, 33, 134, 140

toxin.......26, 29–31, 33, 36, 37, 40, 41,
50, 52, 56, 80–84, 96, 107–109,
111, 113, 114, 123, 134, 140, 141,
147, 149, 150, 153, 154, 163, 164,
166, 168, 170, 171, 173–175, 179,
182, 186, 188–190, 195, 197

toxin exposure.........29, 36, 81, 83, 96,
107, 153

trace minerals...........................93, 178

trans-generational toxins................ 55

trauma............18, 19, 35, 53, 103, 104,
106, 113, 121, 153, 155, 162, 176,
186, 189, 190

Traumatic Brain Injury (TBI).........33,
118, 153

treatment modalities.............109, 117,
120, 129, 132

treatment outcomes....................... 129

treatment protocol................ 124, 125

trembling...148

trichotillomania.............................. 73

triclosan.. 81

trigger 4, 18, 24, 32–36,
43–45, 50, 54, 60, 68, 75, 86, 103,
107, 117, 119–121, 125, 138, 145,
146, 161, 172, 177, 187

trigger foods 86

tryptophan.......................................194

tubulin 48, 156, 200

tumor necrosis factor 32

turmeric 70, 98

TV 21, 80, 88, 160

twirling .... 66. *See also tic*

twitches .... 200. *See also tic*

U

uBiome 96

ultrasounds........................ 33, 54, 153

umeboshi plums 98

underdeveloped airways 122

uneasiness...147

urinary frequency............................ 25

urine tests 92

V

vaccine...143

Valor oil.. 70

Varicella... 47

vegetables.... 85, 88, 98, 140, 185, 196

vetiver oil 97

vibrational therapies.......................142

vinegar..81, 98

vinyl..81, 83

viome 96

viruses.................30, 35, 45, 55, 69, 73,
99, 120, 133, 139, 140, 150, 153,
168, 171, 175, 176, 178, 185, 187,
199, 201

vision impairment...................54, 180

vision therapy.............20, 94, 156–158,
174, 196, 201

visual acuity 94
visual dysfunction 94
visualization 102
visual-motor skills 95
visual stimulation 103, 162
vitamin B$_6$ 42, 164
vitamin C 69, 92, 99, 186
vitamin D.............19, 29, 53, 54, 68, 69,
    83, 84, 92, 96, 110, 111, 202
vitamins................................19, 29, 42,
    53, 54, 61, 64–66, 68, 69, 83, 84, 92,
    96, 99, 110, 111, 164, 179, 184, 186,
    191, 196, 201, 202
vocal tic .... 200. See also tic
VOC paint 81

W

waning of symptoms...................... 131
water filter.. 82
Watkinson, Toby..............12, 136–138,
    141, 142
waxing of symptoms...................... 131
weight gain................................72, 146
weight loss 146
Western blot test 74, 175, 202
Western medicine............7, 44, 64, 75,
    146, 148, 150, 154, 159, 163, 182,
    189, 201, 202
whack-a-mole.................................... 47
wheat................36, 37, 87, 95, 136, 153,
    166, 167
white blood cells...............31, 108, 109,
    169, 198
whole foods 85, 91, 92
WiFi.........33, 34, 54, 80, 114, 123, 137,
    138, 142
WiFi blocking paint........................ 142
William, Anthony............................. 73
winking..................26, 200. See also tic
wireless routers................................ 33
wireless technology........................ 142
writing 19, 95, 153, 158, 197

X

Xanax.. 44
xylene... 110

Y

yeast 42, 61, 96, 144, 154, 166,
    168, 176, 178, 180, 190, 191, 199.
    See also Candida albicans
yeast extract...............................42, 166
yeast infections 154
yoga 99, 186, 201
yogurt 88, 98, 144, 154, 167

Z

zinc...................................53, 90, 93, 178
Zoloft.. 44
zonulin................................. 37, 49, 202
Zyto 50, 74, 77, 159, 202

ABOUT THE AUTHORS

BETH LAMBERT is an author, educator and former healthcare consultant. Beth is the founder and Executive Director of Epidemic Answers, a 501(c)(3) non-profit organization dedicated to reestablishing vibrant health in our children. She is also the creator of The Documenting Hope Project, a multi-year prospective research study and media project that examines the cumulative impact of environmental stressors on children's health. Her first book, *A Compromised Generation: The Epidemic of Chronic Illness in America's Children*, provides a thorough analysis of the origins of this modern health crisis and documents how modifications to environmental and lifestyle factors can profoundly influence health outcomes, including full disease reversal.

MARIA RICKERT HONG is the Media Director for Epidemic Answers and is a Certified Holistic Health Counselor specializing in helping parents make dietary and lifestyle changes for children with Sensory Processing Disorder (SPD), autism, ADHD, allergies, asthma, autoimmune and more. Maria has recovered her sons from SPD, allergies, asthma and acid reflux and is the author of *Almost Autism: Recovering Children from Sensory Processing Disorder, A Reference for Parents and Practitioners*. Maria is a former sell-side Wall Street equity research analyst. Prior to working on Wall Street, she was a marketing specialist for Halliburton in New Orleans, where she also received her MBA in Finance & Strategy from Tulane University.

DR. ROSEANN CAPANNA-HODGE, EdD, LPC, BCN is a Connecticut Certified School Psychologist, a Licensed Professional Counselor (LPC) and a Board Certified Neurofeedback Provider

(BCN), with more than 25 years working with children, teens, adults and parents. She answered her calling to be a psychologist, and currently has private practice offices in Ridgefield and Newtown, CT, where the focus is on neurofeedback, counseling and assessment for a variety of issues and conditions, including specialties in Lyme and PANS/PANDAS. Dr. Roseann is a well-respected BCN practitioner who is a popular and sought after speaker. She serves on the Board of the Northeast Region Biofeedback Society and Lyme Connection Task Force Professional Adviser.

LAUREN LEE STONE, PHD, MS, HHP is a nutritionist and holistic health practitioner who uses BioEnergetic Medicine as a healing modality. Lauren came to BioEnergetic Medicine in the search to heal her own children, and chose to make it her career after experiencing its success first hand. In addition to a BA from Yale University and a PhD from Cornell University, Lauren has a Masters in Human Nutrition from the University of Bridgeport. She also holds an advanced certificate in BioSET, Quantum Reflex Analysis, and is a Certified Holistic Health Practitioner.

JENNIFER GIUSTRA-KOZEK, LPC, NCC, is a board certified licensed psychotherapist with 18 years of clinical experience treating clients with Asperger's, depression, anxiety, OCD and ADHD. She is the author of *Healing without Hurting: Treating ADHD, Apraxia and Autism Spectrum Disorders Naturally and Effectively without Harmful Medication* and the children's book, *A Healthy New Me & ADHD Free.* Jennifer had seen the ADHD/autism epidemic unfold in her own private practice and has watched the harmful impact of medication on many of her young clients. Jennifer earned her Master's Degree in Community Counseling and a Bachelor's Degree in English/Criminal Justice from Western Connecticut State University. She has since become certified in EMDR, reiki and hypnotherapy.

To keep updated and learn more,
visit our websites at
www.BrainUnderAttack.com and
www.EpidemicAnswers.org

Made in the USA
Middletown, DE
02 January 2023

20784369R00142